108 Years

A Korean Way of Health

Young Ahn Kwon

Lloyd Sparks

For my family

Contents

Co-Author's Preface	1
Preface by Master Jerry O'Donoghue	4
Foreword	6
Chapter 1 – Coming to America	11
Chapter 2 – My Life Plan	22
Chapter 3 - Daily Habits That Lead to Health	25
Chapter 4 – Food and Water	49
Chapter 5 – Lessons from a Long Life	54
Chapter 6 – Family Values	58
Chapter 7 – Taekwondo	66
Chapter 8 – Hokwondo	72
Chapter 9 – Decide Now	74
Korean Terms	76
About the Authors	77

Co-Author's Preface

The first thing you notice about Grandmaster Kwon is how fit he is. At seventy, he is trim, energetic, and impressively flexible.

The second thing is his smile. *Kwan Jang Nim,* (Grandmaster, in Korean) as he is addressed by his students, is infectiously optimistic. Just being in the same room with him will brighten anyone's day.

I met Grandmaster Kwon quite by accident in 2009. A friend informed me she was testing for Black Belt in Taekwondo along with her two teenage children and she invited me to attend the ceremony. I had no particular interest in Taekwondo and wasn't looking to study another martial art. I came out of courtesy to my friend.

What I saw changed my life.

Here was a martial arts academy nestled in a small town in Massachusetts that was unlike any other I had visited in my five decades since Bruce Lee first sparked my adolescent interest in the Asian fighting arts. For one thing, it was a family-centered *dojang* (martial arts training school). It didn't emphasize self-defense, competition, and fighting, although those are integral elements. Grandmaster Kwon was running a martial arts-based family fitness organization of his own creation based on the ancient Korean fighting art of Taekwondo.

The students were smiling, having fun and, most remarkably, many were there as families. The students ranged from small children to adults in their sixties. The instructors were professional but kind. The air was punctuated with shouts of "high five!" and "good job!" The stern and harsh drill sergeant-like demeanor of so many martial arts instructors was absent. This was all the more remarkable in that the instructors themselves were mostly Korean and all impressively skilled.

Grandmaster Kwon was by far the most skilled of all. Pictures of his more impressive feats decorate the corridor. (In one, he is breaking four one-inch pine boards suspended freely from one hand with a fist while doing the splits balanced on a couple of chairs.) The opportunity to study at the feet (so to speak) of a 9th dan grandmaster (there is no 10th dan level) was too good an opportunity to pass up, so I joined in 2009 as a humble white belt.

What I did not know at the time, and learned as I trained faithfully twice a week over the ensuing years, was that Grandmaster Kwon was also trained in the traditional healing arts of Korea. I learned of his skill through my own misfortune when in 2014 I was diagnosed with cancer.

While I was undergoing conventional treatment for the disease, *Kwan Jang Nim* took a compassionate interest in my case and offered his services. After a long and detailed interview, which involved painstakingly looking up all of the relevant medical terms in a dictionary, he gave me his recommendation, which I took to heart.

I was to do a 9-week purifying and rejuvenating diet along with incorporating several daily physical practices of self-massage and exercise. From a conventional Western medical point of view, my prognosis was serious. I had less than 40 percent chance I would survive even two years. As a trained physician myself, I chose to undergo the conventional treatments I know and trust, but also followed *Kwan Jang Nim's* regimen.

Today I am cancer-free.

Grandmaster Kwon's personal example is the best proof of the value of what you will find in this book. Although seventy at this writing, he is the fittest man I know out of a host of fit, elderly individuals. Fitness is my hobby; it is *Kwan Jang Nim's* life.

It is very difficult to convey the voice of the grandmaster, loved by so many as by me. English is not his native language and he is at his best when he can show what he wants to communicate. Much of what he has to say is highly detailed and technical. I've worked hard with the help of his children, Masters Jayne and Greg, to capture the precise meaning of what he wants to convey. I'm also indebted to his students of many years who know him best for their help. I have resisted inserting my opinions and interpretations into his message as much as possible. When I think there is some additional understanding to be had from medical science or believe that some clarification might be helpful, I've tried to make it clear that they are my own comments.

I've endeavored to stand aside and let Grandmaster Kwon say everything his way. Nevertheless, I'm afraid my voice will come through the text, but it can't be helped. Please be assured that the English text may sound like me, his co-author, but the message is entirely his.

This does not excuse me from unintentional inaccuracies that the careful reader is sure to uncover. For those shortcomings, I apologize in advance and take full responsibility.

This is a singularly unique work. I know of no popular book on a martial arts-based Korean health system available in English. Even if there were stacks of them, Grandmaster Kwon's book would still stand as a valuable contribution to the health and well-being of the inhabitants of this planet. Early in our conversations about writing the book, *Kwan Jang Nim* said, "There are too many hospitals! More full hospitals than when I came to this country over 30 years ago. Why?" His answer to his own rhetorical question was that people do not take care of themselves.

This book is about taking care of ourselves.

Kwan Jang Nim makes the argument that we must take care of others first, then ourselves. We are all connected. There is no individual health that does not affect the health of everyone else. In interviewing my fellow disciples for this book, I found case after case of people turning their health around for the better because of the inspiration and the instruction of the grandmaster.

Conversely, there is no illness that does not affect us all, either. This is a very relevant conversation today as the debate over healthcare simmers in the halls of government and the pages of Facebook. Should we trust the government or private industry to guarantee health to all citizens? Grandmaster Kwon would say, "No!"

Your health is your responsibility; it comes from within you.

So does your happiness. As you will see as you read, all happiness and health start with your mental attitude. From that come right actions (through the instruction of wise teachers) which bloom into health-supporting habits that lead to happiness and fitness long into old age.

"Very, very basic; very, very small," he said over and over again as he described to me the details of actions and habits that will lead to health and happiness. Little thoughts and actions matter. From tiny acorns grow mighty oaks.

Throughout the book you, dear reader, will catch whiffs of ancient Asian concepts like "karma" and "chi." I've chosen to use the grandmaster's words and keep to his simple English terminology as much as possible. It would be an inexcusable injustice to render his teaching into just another book about yoga or Buddhist meditation.

Grandmaster Kwon's story is unique and deserves to be told the way he tells it.

~ Lloyd Sparks, MD
3rd Dan Black Belt

Preface by Master Jerry O'Donoghue

I have been a student of Grandmaster Kwon for over ten years now. What can I say about Kwanjangnim that hasn't already been said? The truth is, I can't. I can only give you a glimpse into my own experience, about the man I have come to know and trust.

Trust is the key word. I don't use it lightly.

Everyone who meets Kwanjangnim will pick up on the fact that he is not the kind of person you meet every day. His passion for life and helping others is extraordinary, and absolutely genuine. Not only for his many students, but many people going through a tough time in their life outside of martial arts altogether.

I have learned so much about life in general from Kwanjangnim. Everything from eating a healthy diet, a great and easy way to naturally clean out the toxins from my system, to the best way to exercise as my body is getting older. Some may be skeptical, given that I'm one of his students. I assure you I have tried everything myself that Kwanjangnim has taught us all in class, and have found out, first hand, the benefits they have. As a young fella, turning fifty in a few months, I am in better physical and mental health than most people twenty years younger that I work with. That feels good.

Simple things, like stretching before getting out of bed in the morning. Since our bodies take a while to wake up, light stretching in a warm and comfortable bed helps the body to wake up slowly while loosening up joints before gravity takes hold of us. I used to, very painfully, make my way to the shower like an old man from many years of working in construction, and sport-related injuries. Everything from ruptured Achilles tendons to having one of many herniated discs come out during the night. This stretching is invaluable for anyone like me.

About five years ago, I had a heart attack. The medical specialists put it down to stress. Against Kwanjangnim's advice, I took a break from Taekwondo. I realized my mistake sooner rather than later, thank God. He was right, taking class at my own pace really helped with stress, and overall health.

One evening before class I was having chest pain. I can remember it like it was yesterday. Kwanjangnim brought me into his office and after making sure I was in no danger, started working on pressure points and explaining what he was doing and how it works. Long story short, the pain subsided, and I had very enjoyable class. I use what he taught me often. That is what Kwanjangnim is well known for, sharing his knowledge and his own life experiences with us simply makes him happy. That's what makes him tick.

Our beautiful daughter has benefited very much from getting to know Kwanjangnim also. She has ADD, SID, PDD, Asperger's, and a host of problems that make everyday life a challenge. Kwanjangnim has influenced her in a very positive way. He has earned her trust, not an easy thing to do, I can assure you. She takes all the information Kwanjangnim shares with us, on a weekly basis, and puts them to practice herself outside of the school. She has really come into her own over the last few years. Going to class and meeting Kwanjangnim is definitely the high point in her week. She's always asking, "when are we going to class again?"

The information that Kwanjangnim imparts to everyone, in this book, is quite simply to enrich everyone's life, so we can grow old gracefully, healthier, and hopefully happier. When you try these techniques, you will be pleasantly surprised. I could go on forever, but I think you get the picture. Simply, my life has been enriched for getting to know this unique person, Grandmaster Kwon.

~ Master Jerry O'Donoghue
5th Dan Black Belt

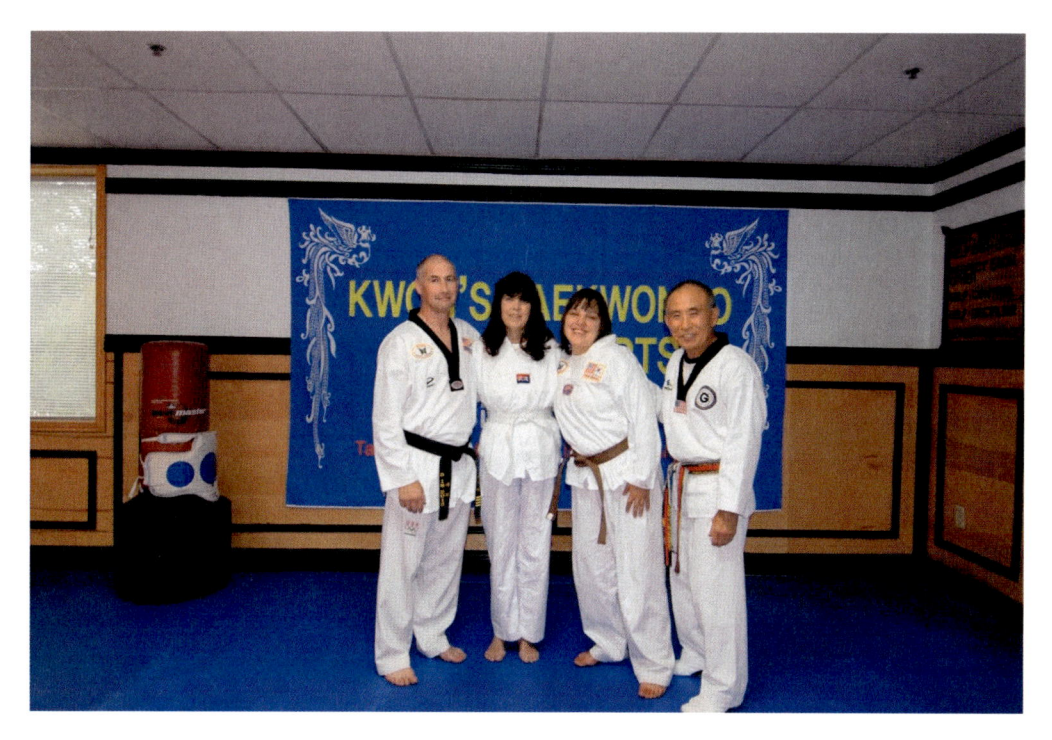

Master Jerry O'Donoghue with wife, daughter, and Grandmaster Kwon

Foreword

"I have learned so much about training and good health from Grandmaster Kwon...chief among them is the new definition of healthy that I've gained by not only listening carefully to his recommendations and experiences, but by finding the right combination of exercise, nutrition, and rest for myself. I now firmly believe, as he says, that anyone can achieve the top 5% of good health and that it can be fun getting there."

~ Mark Fortune
3rd Dan Black Belt

"One of the reasons I think he has been such a great leader is the fact that he leads by example. My daughter started practicing Taekwondo with Grandmaster Kwon around five years ago and he motivated me to start practicing the discipline. I'm so happy I decided to start practicing. As a physician, I know how important it is to keep your body and mental health in good shape. He has dedicated his whole life to practice and development of martial arts and has done with so much passion that is really inspiring."

~ Jose R. Gutierrez, MD

There are too many hospitals. Too many *full* hospitals. It seems like there are many more than when I came to this country 30 years ago. More than in the past. Why?

People don't take care of themselves. They're too busy, they neglect themselves, they do too many small, bad things which become habits and result in bad energy.

As I begin this book – a collection of the advice I would give to anyone who wants to stay fit and healthy for 108 years – it is summer. It is the time when people start doing things to make themselves look better on the outside. They get a tan. They put on makeup. They go to the gym to lose weight and build muscle. Everybody works on the outside.

Nobody works on the inside!

This book was not written overnight. It is the product of many years of experience, of making notes of ideas from the heart. It is intended to give a little push to those who need hope and confidence in their path to health and to provide guidance for self-help and care.

I know many people with health issues. I am writing this book to help others, but it also recharges me at my age of 70. It is the small light from a candle to help you see. It is like a root that can grow into a big tree.

In Korean we say, "It will happen only if you try." Too many people say, "I can't do it." Their minds are too tight. They need to open up. This book is like a key that opens the door. Nobody can turn the key for you.

Just like the candle in which heat and light cannot be separated, the mental cannot be separated from the physical. You must take care for your health your whole life. Do the healthy practices over and over. Just like reading a book over and over, gradually you will see and understand more and more. And the healthy practices are free! Isn't this the best way? Simple, easy, and can be done anywhere and without harmful side effects.

We live in a free country. Why keep a closed mind? Start small. Don't start with high expectations. Don't overthink your problems. Keep things basic. Let the bad energy out and the good energy in by keeping your mind open.

There was a study done of 12 people with cancer. Six were given chemotherapy and six were given only placebo. But all 12 reacted as if they had the chemo. Their hair fell out. In six of these patients, their expectations alone made their bodies react as if they were getting chemotherapeutic drugs.

Your mental attitude affects your physical health. Positive expectations are very important. The mental – how you think about things – plays a huge part in your wellness. You must focus to make the mental and physical become one.

If you lack health, you can't enjoy this beautiful world. Do simple exercises you can do for free without help.

Beauty

The prettiest flower is a happy face, and a happy face is truly like a flower. It blooms from the inside. No one picks a flower and just sticks it onto a stem; the flower grows out of the inner goodness of the seed, taking energy from the sun, the air, and the soil.

Pick a flower and it will fade. Feed a flower and it will stay fresh and beautiful.

A beautiful flower grows through hard times – rain, wind, frost, and such. Then it gives happiness to others by sharing its beauty. Even if you grow up in a tough environment or with a handicap, don't lose hope. Keep a strong mind and body.

We shape our lives with the good and bad energy we move in ourselves, mental and physical. Don't be a fish in a bowl! Small worlds are for closed minds. Jump out of the bowl and discover the ocean! It all starts with a decision. Be a force for good! Start today!

"Grandmaster Kwon says learning should be fun and creates an idyllic atmosphere by inviting parents, friends, irrespective of athletic ability. He says we should always bring happiness to ourselves and always smile. I have tried it out and it really works. In fact, research shows that smiling helps us live longer and happier. It activates one's qi."

~ Jonathan Kasule
2nd Dan Black Belt

Happiness

You create your own happiness or sadness. It is not given to you by others. If health is your first priority, everything else will succeed. If it isn't, nothing will. Making money should never come before staying healthy.

Helping people makes you happy and keeps good energy flowing. If you are thirsty and you give water to a thirsty man, you feel better, too. If you have good things inside yourself – love, wisdom, advice – share them with others. By sharing them, you will improve your own health. If you keep everything to yourself and hold them inside, it will lead to bad health and physical deterioration.

Sharing of yourself is more meaningful and valuable than money or material goods. Lose your greed and overcome possessiveness. Selfishness leads to bad energy and bad health. When you help people, it comes back to you. First help others, then yourself. Be kind to one another. A smile adds three minutes to your life. Each angry face takes away nine minutes.

Share knowledge and experience with others. That's what this book is all about, for the next generation. Following health leads people in a good path. When people are born, they are soft but become stiff and dry as they age. Just as plants start out young and green with water, they end up dry and brittle at the end.

Selfishness is hard and dry. It leads to early death. Open-mindedness is flexibility and keeps you young. The key to a longer life is flexibility, sharing, and helping others. Even keeping a pet counts as caring for others.

Why do you want to live a longer life? If you live only for yourself, your life will have no meaning. Nothing of yourself will live on after you are gone. But if you share, your life will live on through others.

A Life Plan

"Grandmaster Kwon is the toughest trainer I ever had. Even the other Korean instructors fear him."

~ Grandmaster Michael Couhie

The world is getting easier, resulting in lazier habits. We don't have to work as hard as we used to. But nothing of value is created without hard work and commitment. If you want to be happy and healthy, you must plan for it and then carry out the plan no matter what.

Make a promise to yourself to make a life plan and keep it. If you do not keep promises to yourself, you will not keep promises to others and your reputation will suffer. Unkept promises will bother you inside. This is the beginning of decline of health.

If you don't have a life plan, you won't know whether you're are succeeding or not. If you have a plan, you can check to see whether your life is going well and correct it when it isn't. From time to time, stop and check in with yourself. Who am I? Where am I on my life path? Readjust and recharge your energy.

Most people don't even know they have a problem. "No problem" is the problem!

All plans start out happy, then become difficult. Life is full of ups and downs. Don't quit in the middle of your plan. Giving up leads to bad energy and decline in health.

"Being active and exercising are very important parts of maintaining a healthy lifestyle. As a parent, I found it was difficult to find time for me to exercise because I was constantly taking my sons to all of their activities. Taekwondo is the way that I am able to balance family time and exercise. Taekwondo has allowed us to spend time together as a family exercising, having fun, and enjoying family time. We are fortunate to have been able to train in a welcoming environment at Kwon's Taekwondo with Grandmaster Kwon and the other masters and instructors. This past spring my youngest son and I earned our first-degree black belts and my oldest son earned his third-degree black belt. We accomplished this together as a family and we are looking forward to continuing our training with Grandmaster Kwon".

~ Shelby, Joshua, and Andrew Gauvin
Black Belt Family

Your Thought Life and Mental Attitude

Think hard about your plan. Start with a good mental attitude. Mental comes before physical. Small things matter. Everyone is born with 108 years of potential life energy. Living long and healthy depends on your attitude and your thoughts which lead to actions. Small, small actions lead to strong habits and big results.

"I work as a kindergarten teacher. Grandmaster Kwon sends an instructor down once or twice a week to instill all these positive traits in small children. They get an early taste of taking care of their bodies, protecting themselves, discipline, and perseverance.

I have seen him encourage a child with autism who earned her black belt under his guidance. I have seen him be a positive male role model for children without fathers. He explains the difference between right and wrong and the children respect him. He teaches them about respectful behavior as well as protecting themselves which is very much appreciated by many moms.

Grandmaster Kwon is so very helpful to me in my own personal life. I have celiac disease and type-2 diabetes. My memory is another thing that I feel is slipping away from me as I get a little older. I have added Taekwondo to my workout regimen hoping to give a boost to my already compromised health. He sat me down and gave me some helpful food tips to help with my health and I followed his directions.

One day he was speaking to me and another mom when we said we wish we had started practicing Taekwondo when we were young. He told us that it is never too late to start Taekwondo and it's better to start now than never. I'm currently a 46-year-old blue belt, but I intend on persevering over my age, my illnesses, my lack of memory, and any other obstacle until I get my black belt. I intend to be the best person I can, thanks to Grandmaster Kwon."

~ Nancy Martin-Roque
Blue Belt

The Five Divisions of Life

Life is separated into five divisions:

0 – 24 years: These are the growing years from baby to college student. They are a time for learning and being cared for by parents, family, and teachers. If you think of your life like sports, this is when you play for fun and go to the pre-season tryouts.

25 – 45 years: This is the first phase of adulthood. It is a time of high energy, excitement, and optimism. It is when you make your big decisions about your career and life partner. In sports, this period is like the draft when players go from being amateurs to professionals.

46 – 65 years: These are the middle years of the productive phase of adulthood, a time of steady growth and production. You build your career, your home, and your family in these years. It is the playing season of your life.

66 – 85 years: This is the final peak phase, the culmination of your life's work and a time of intense challenge to finish the job. You are now in the championships, the Super Bowl of life.

86 – 108 years: These are the years of old age, of steady continuity, and a time for contemplation. It is a time for coaching young players and watching the other teams play.

Health is not just for the young. We need energy in our older years to not give up right when our lives are coming to their peaks. We need energy to enjoy life and appreciate the good things we have built. People only realize how important health is when they lose it and wind up in the hospital.

Just like we don't see the electricity that powers our lights, we don't see our inner energy. But it is just as real. You can feel it! You can feel how it flows, where it is blocked, and how it connects you to others.

Energy is life!

Chapter 1 – Coming to America

"One of the Korean grandmasters told me, 'We lost a national treasure when Grandmaster Kwon left for America'."

~ Grandmaster Michael Couhie

"I started Tae Kwon Do a lot later in life than most do. I was active in my youth and in college but then I got married and had two sons. My focus was on things other than myself. So, when the opportunity to try this martial art presented itself I was committed but very out of shape. Simply running around the room made me breathe very heavy. I consider myself very fortunate indeed to have found Grandmaster Kwon and his wonderful school when I did. I found a man who generously shares his knowledge, his time, and his love of Tae Kwon Do with all who ask for it. He does not judge you against some artificial standard but instead he asks only that you do the very best that you can. Naturally, this makes you try all the harder to honor him and his school. His encouragement, faith in me and friendship mean everything, and I would have been much poorer if we had not met."

~ Master Robin Zukowski
5th Dan Black Belt

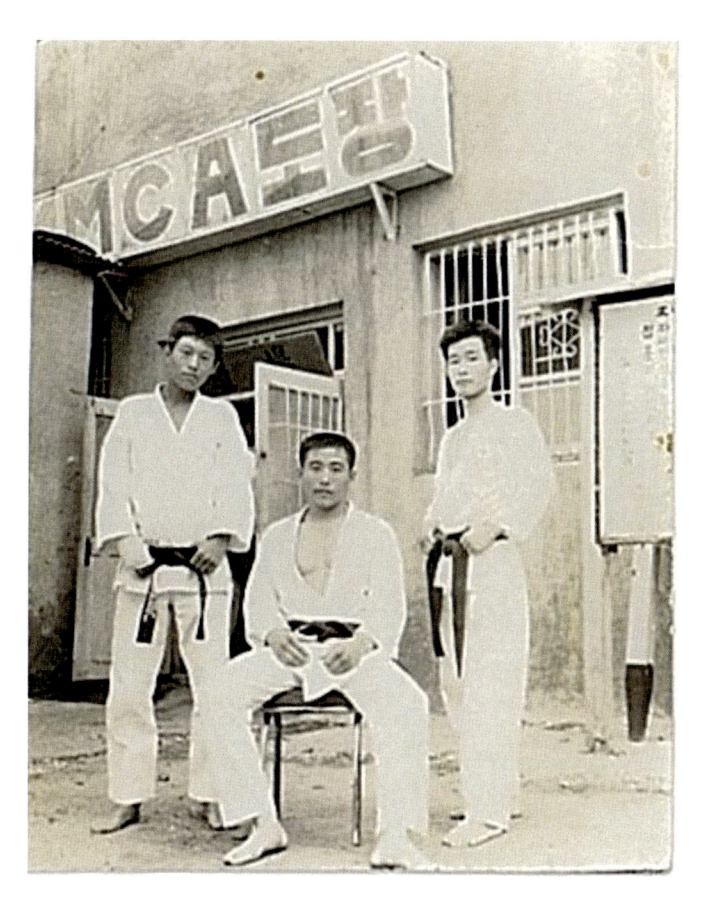

Training (seated, center) at the YMCA dojang in 1964 as 2nd Dan Black Belt

I came to this country for a ten-day Taekwondo exhibition and stayed for the rest of my life.

In 1987, I had been running a Taekwondo school in Korea along with a private practice in acupuncture for about 15 years. The Korean Taekwondo Association asked me to take part in a goodwill tour to the United States as part of a Taekwondo demonstration team.

It was a wonderful experience. We performed in such famous cities as San Francisco and New Orleans and the ten days went by very fast. We were all on three-month visas, so when the tour was over, most of us stayed to see more of America and visit friends and relatives.

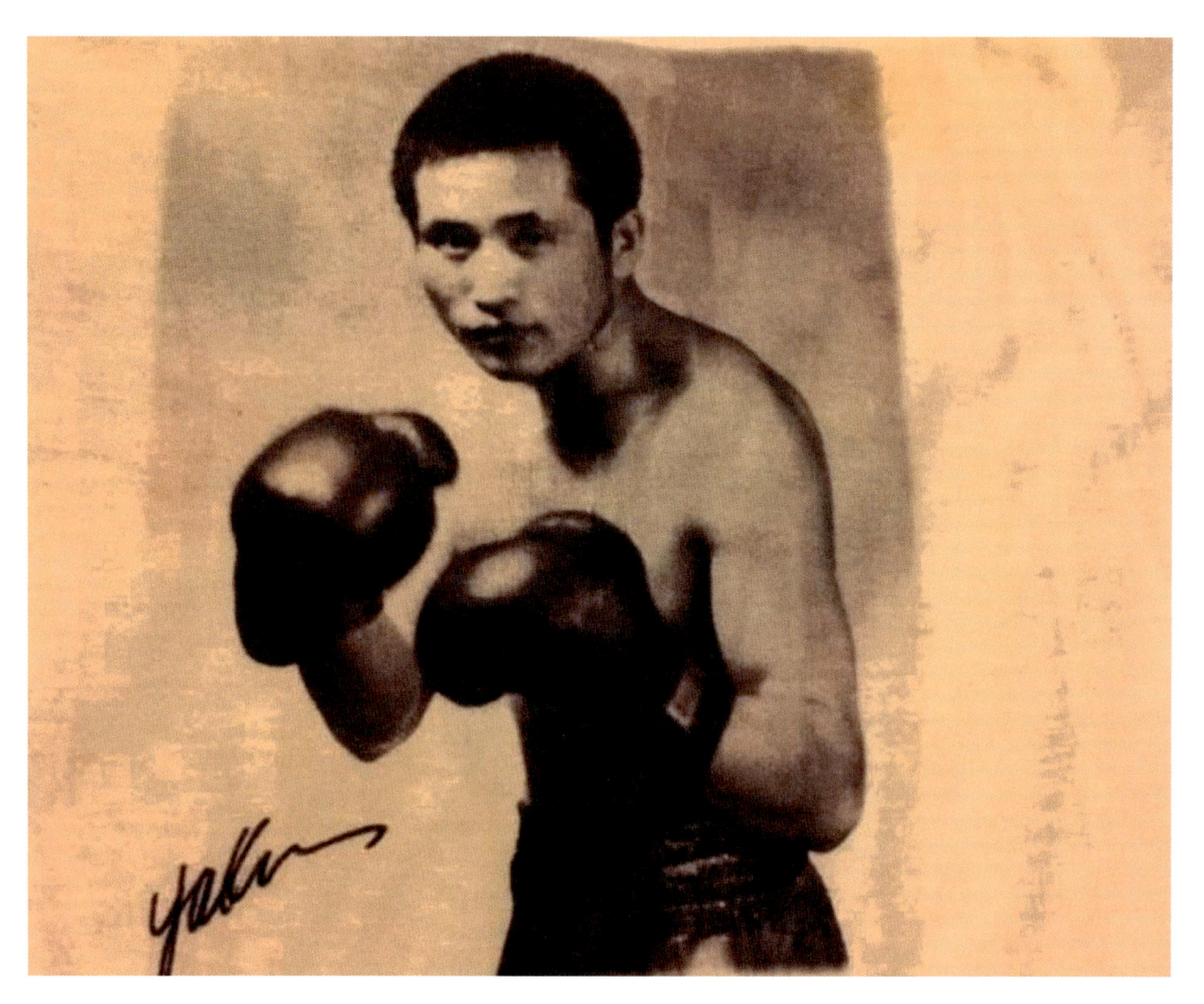

Grandmaster Kwon as a young kick boxer

A close friend of mine in Korea had a brother who ran a Taekwondo school in Lawrence, Massachusetts, not far from Boston. I decided to visit him. After a few days, I realized how much I loved America! Even though I spoke almost no English and didn't have much money, I was sure this was the place I should stay and build a life.

I could work teaching at my friend's school and certainly find some other work to do in the Korean community. My school and acupuncture practice in Korea were in the hands of a capable assistant manager, so there was no reason not to try to stay.

I immediately found an immigration attorney and began the process of applying for a permanent visa. Because both martial arts teacher and acupuncturist are skills in demand, I could apply for a visa on that basis. I soon received permission to stay for three years.

The Medicine Man

At a tournament I attended in 1987, one of the contestants suffered a broken nose. Such an injury is not rare in Taekwondo and I knew how to fix it, but everyone said not to touch the injured man for of fear of being sued. I fixed it anyway, then put ice on it until the paramedics arrived. For an injury like this, you must first reset the broken bone before the swelling starts. Fix first, then ice. Otherwise it won't heal after the swelling comes.

The story was written up in the local newspaper and I became known as "the medicine man."

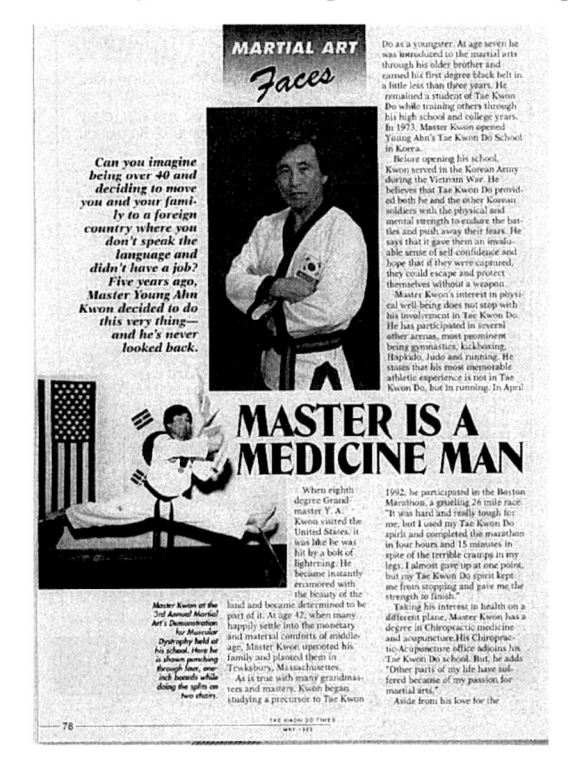

During that time, I visited the Korean community outside of Ft. Devens in the little town of Ayer. There are communities of foreigners near most US military bases because American servicemen often bring home foreign wives – German, Japanese, Filipino, Vietnamese, Thai, and Korean, to mention only a few.

I found a room for rent with a Korean lady whose husband was American. She wanted $700 a month, but that was a lot. I offered $500, but she said no. She had a painful shoulder, which I treated with acupuncture, so eventually she let me stay for $600, but that was an exceptional case. She could have gotten $700 from someone else.

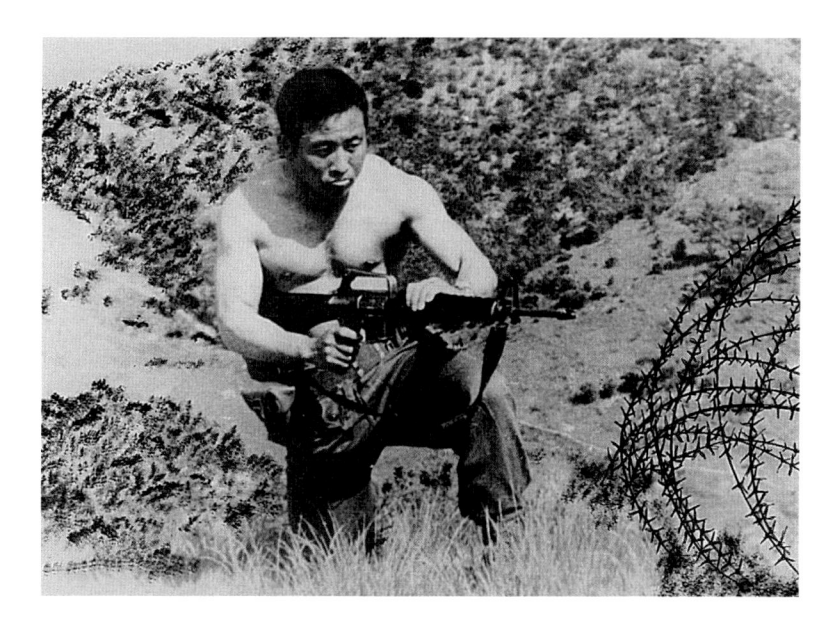

Grandmaster Kwon as a young ROK Marine commando

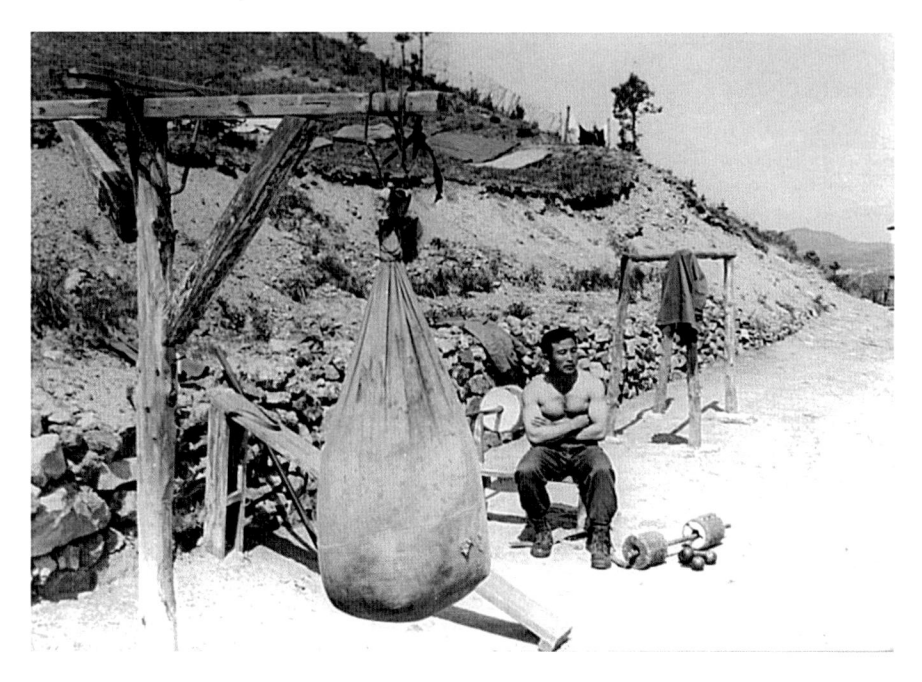

Physical training was an important part of the ROK Marine Corps

Her husband introduced me to one of the officers on base at Ft. Devens, and soon I was teaching martial arts to the soldiers of the American Special Forces. I had served in Special Operations in the South Korean Marines, so I had a very good relationship with the Americans, even though I had to use a translator to teach. It didn't matter. Taekwondo is about action and Green Berets are action people.

I used to go to the park to run and work out for an hour every day. One Sunday, I was feeling a little more tired than usual, so I came home early. It was a good thing I did! As I walked in the door, I heard the landlady screaming "Help me!" She had had a stroke and half her body was paralyzed with her arms twisted at an odd angle.

I treated her with acupuncture and within half an hour, the twists were gone. They medevacked her to Worcester hospital by helicopter where she received excellent medical care. One month later she was completely well.

Most strokes do not recover 100%, but she did. She called me every week after that and would often bring by some food to say thanks. She is still alive, in her 80s.

Timing is Everything

I tell this story to illustrate that good timing is everything in life. The chance that she would rent to me for $600, that I would have the skills to treat her, that I would come home just at the right time, all had to be in place for her to recover from her stroke. Otherwise, she might have died or been paralyzed for life.

A Boston newspaper wrote up the story, again calling me "the medicine man," so I gained a little more popularity.

After three years, I qualified for a Green Card and could start my own business. I was very excited, even though many people tried to talk me out of it. I was renting too much space, they said. My English wasn't good enough, they said. I would never get enough students to cover the expenses, they said. But I believed the school would be a success with all my heart. It took me over a year to break even, but eventually we thrived and have been in operation at the same location now for almost 30 years!

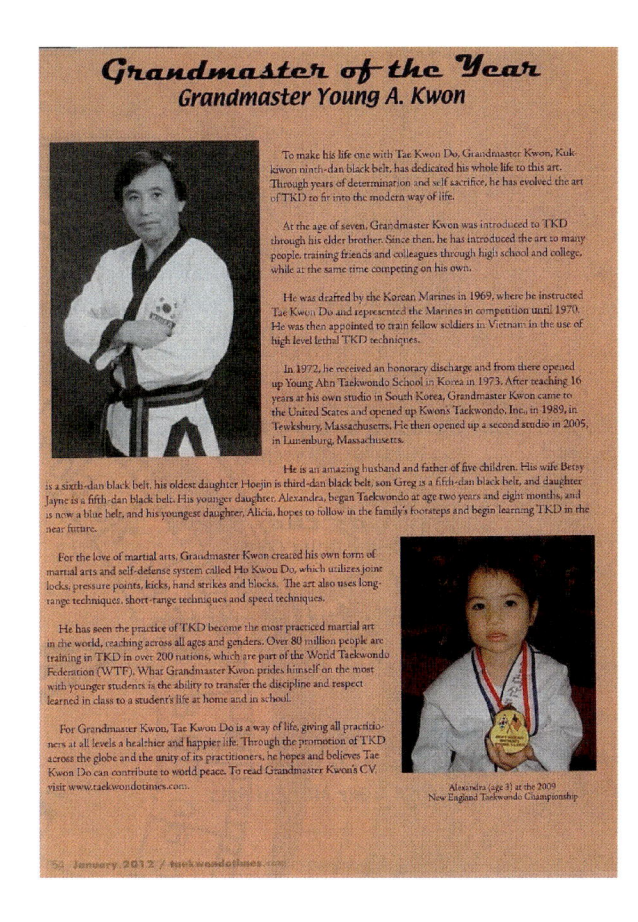

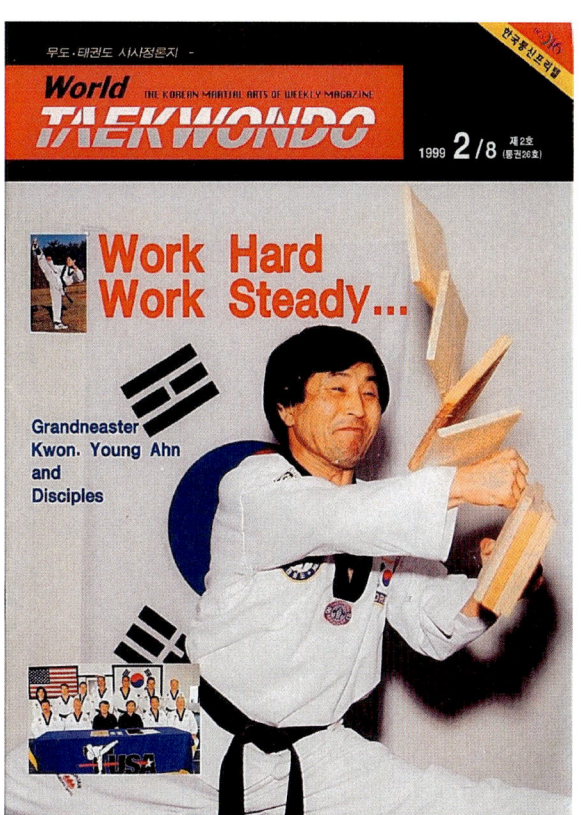

"I started learning martial arts at age 13. In college, I looked for a good school taught by a grandmaster from Korea. Although there are many Taekwondo schools in Massachusetts, I used to drive 18 miles three to five times a week from Boston to train at Grandmaster Kwon's school. During the first year, I brought some friends to watch class and they immediately signed up. There was no pressure to enroll. Grandmaster Kwon's advice was just to try to do your best, help each other, and never give up. After 17 years and earning my 5th dan (master level) Black Belt, I am still coming to class to train and help train others."

~ Master Tae W. Kim
5th Dan Black Belt

(Next page) Master Betsy Kwon and Grandmaster Young A. Kwon - Taekwondo demonstration to benefit the fundraiser for Muscular Dystrophy Association

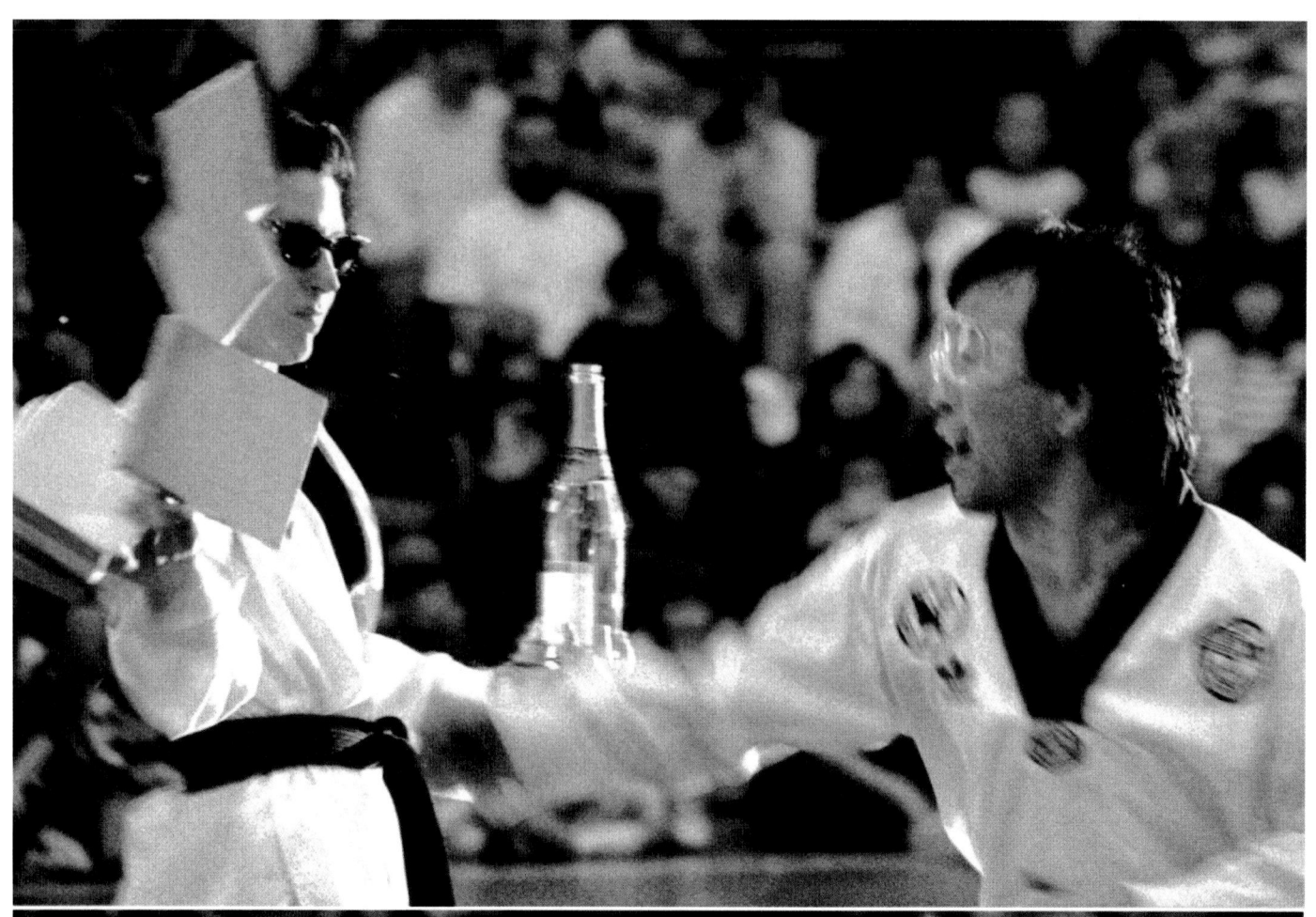

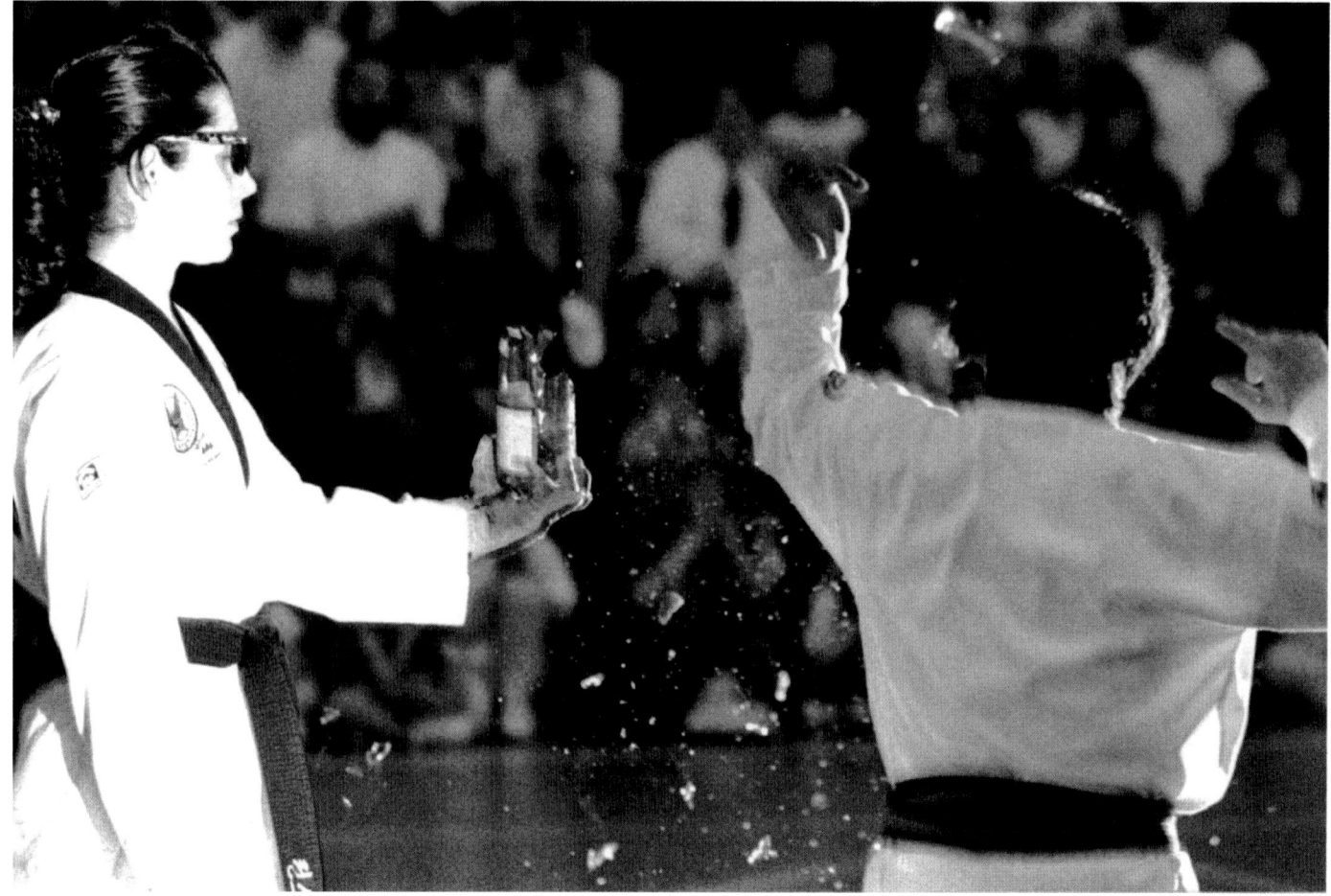

The Boston Marathon

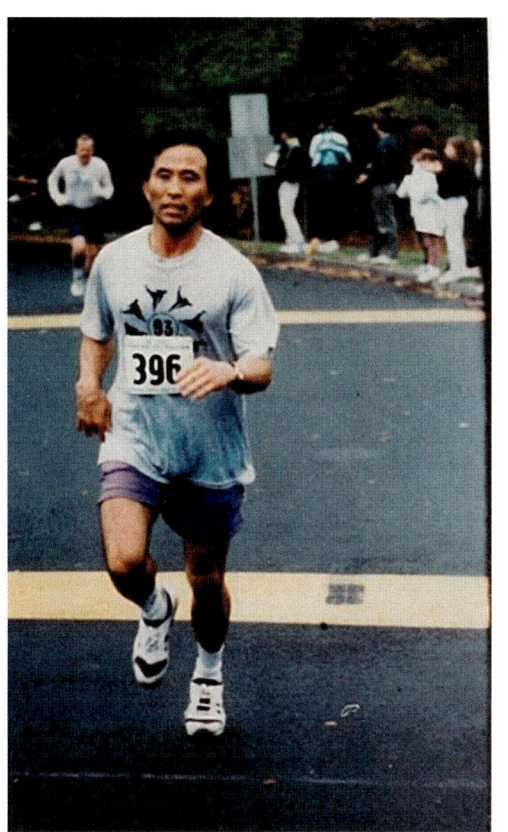

While teaching at my new *dojang* (school), I met a man who worked at the local hardware store. He was a distance runner and told me about the Boston marathon he would be running in. I like to run, so I agreed to train with him and enter the famous race.

We trained regularly at the Tewksbury High School track and by the day of the race, we were ready! My friend and his colleagues were experienced marathoners, but this was my first one. Before long, they were far ahead of me.

I kept on at my pace and soon discovered that I had made a serious mistake in training. The high school track is flat, but the Boston marathon is full of hills. Some of them are really hard! At about mile 18, I began to feel faint. I saw stars and had to stop before I lost consciousness and fell over.

I had brought my acupuncture needles with me in a little pack, so I took them out and treated myself to regain energy. The paramedics came to check me out, but I assured them I was fine and wished to continue the race.

I eventually finished with a time of over four hours. My friends finished almost an hour quicker than me, but they were still waiting for me at the finish line! I apologized for being so slow, but they were not the least bit angry and congratulated me for finishing.

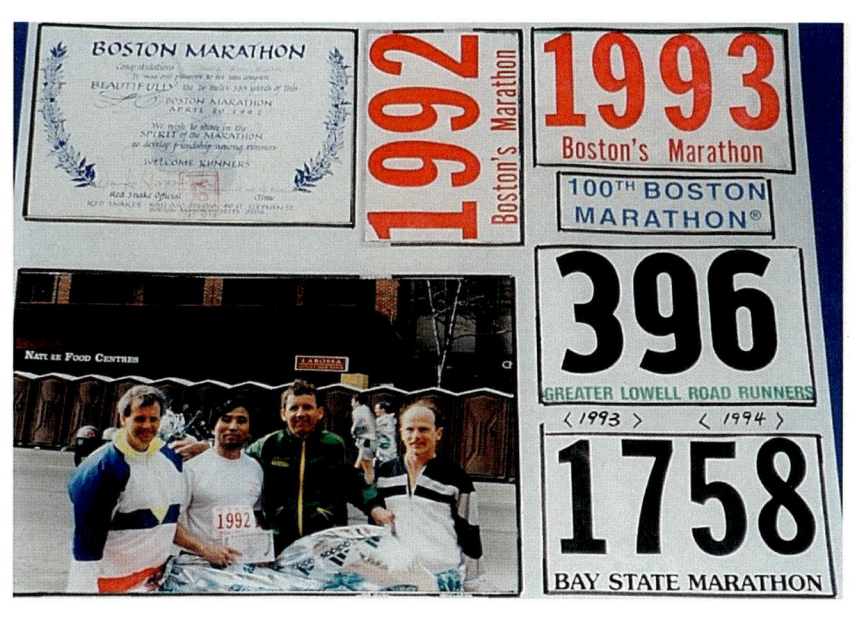

Later, *Taekwondo Times* wrote up an article about my experience, again calling me "the medicine man."

I have since completed seven marathons and my best times are under four hours. But I do not recommend running for exercise unless you really like it. It takes a long, long time to train for endurance events like marathons. You must run hundreds of miles just to be ready for a 26-mile race. To train for a marathon requires dedication and discipline. You spend hour after hour just picking your feet up and putting them down on the pavement.

Right from the beginning, I treated people with acupuncture and chiropractic[1] like I did in Korea. There was a big demand for my services in the Korean community. I also encountered injuries and illness at my school

---

[1] The purely American discipline of chiropractic, invented in 1895, is based on finding and reducing subluxations (minor displacements) of the vertebrae in order to relieve pressure on nerves. The origin of the word is Greek and means "to do by hand" or "to manipulate." Chiropractic, as Grandmaster Kwon uses the term, involves manual therapy beyond just manipulating the

which I knew 100% how to treat. I was happy to offer my skills where ever I could, but I learned that I would need a license to practice acupuncture or chiropractic in any state of the United States.

It is a moral dilemma when you know how to treat a patient but have to withhold treatment because you don't have a license. There are the so-called "Good Samaritan" laws that protect people who try to help but aren't licensed. But it seemed best to get a license if I wanted to continue to practice without worrying about getting sued.

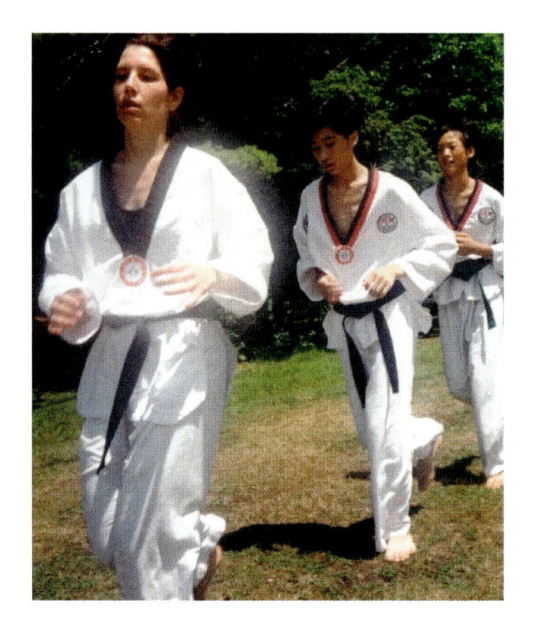

First from left: Master Betsy Kwon

Third from left: Master Greg Kwon

1993 White Mountain spring training, running barefoot.

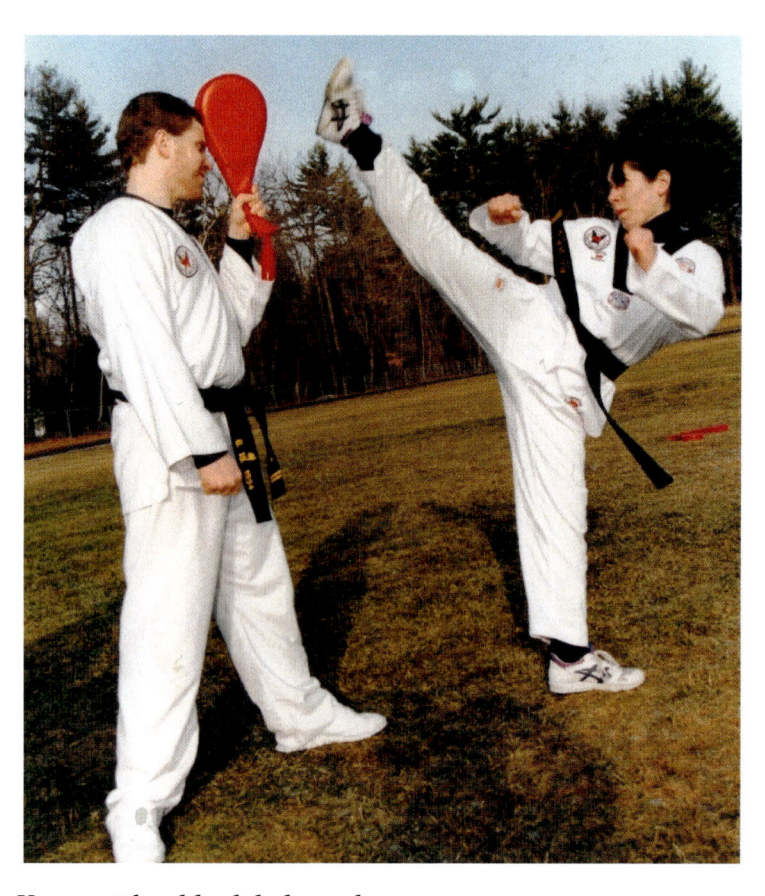

Master Betsy Kwon with a black belt student

spine.

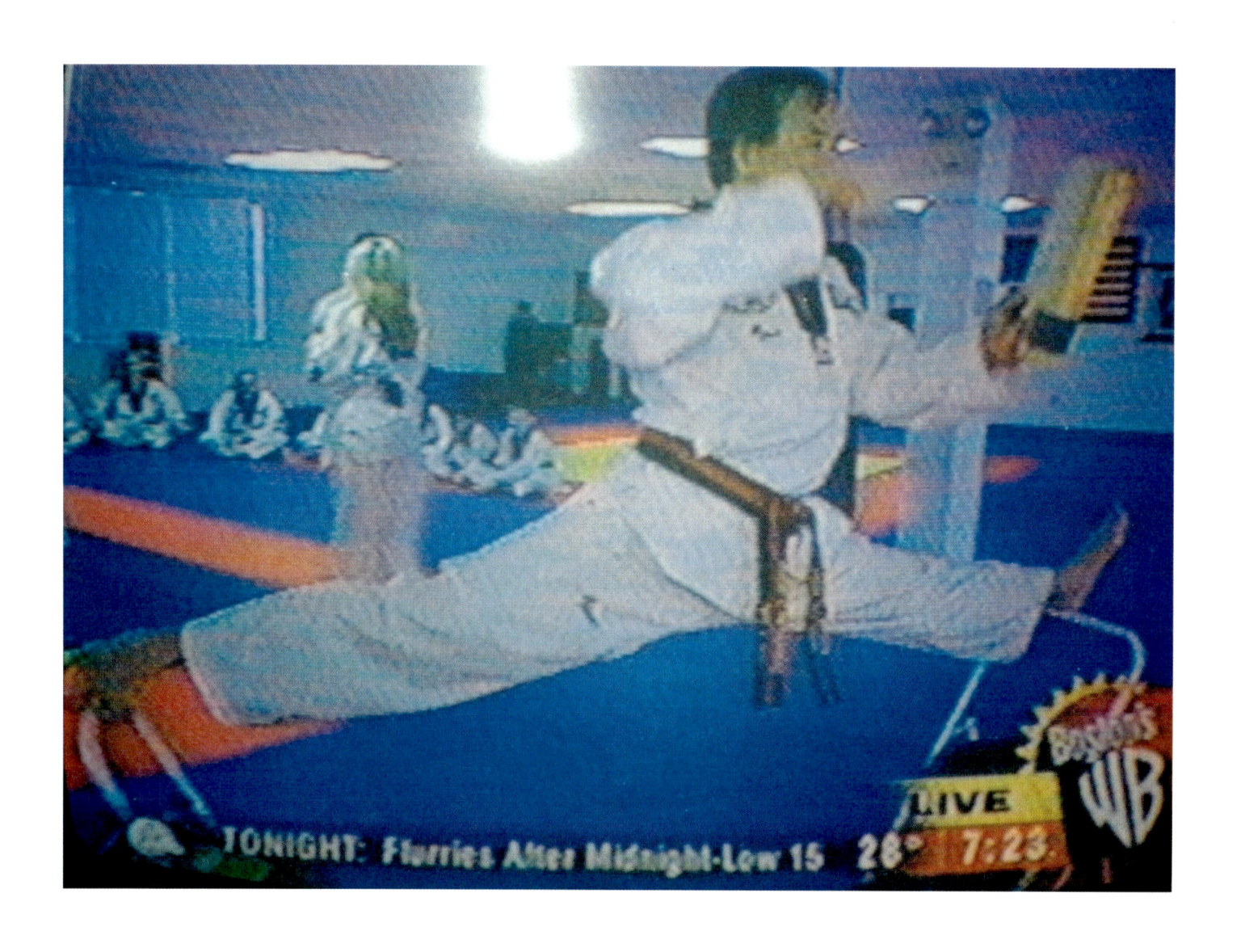

Grandmaster Kwon appeared in a Taekwondo demonstration on WB Channel 56

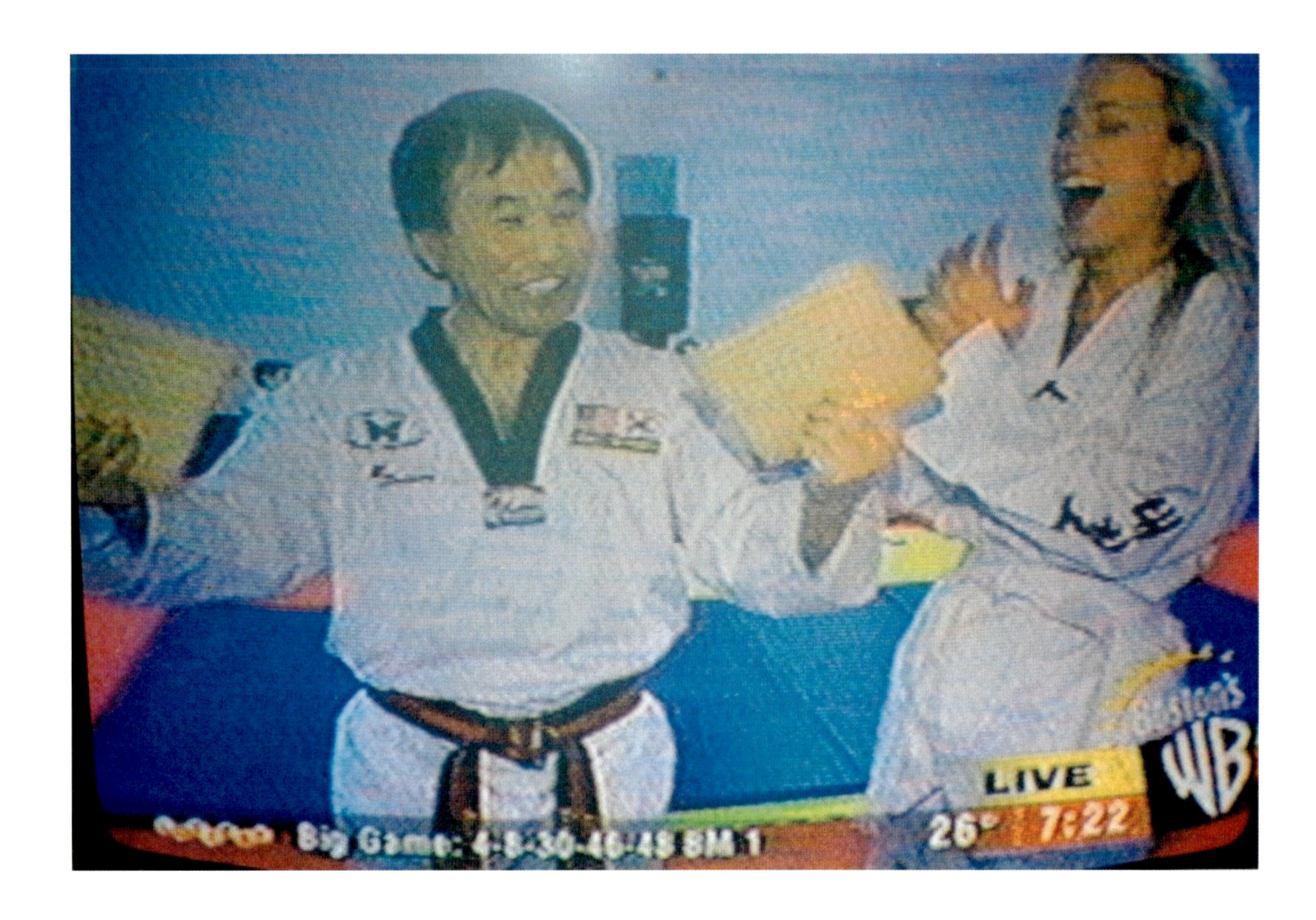

Healing as a Moral Obligation

The tests for acupuncture and chiropractic licenses are very complex and all in English. I have the courage to do very dangerous things as a Korean Marine and as a martial arts fighter. But just to answer the phone in English when I first started out was the scariest thing I have ever done in my life! The idea of studying English for years just to pass a test in acupuncture seemed like too much work for something that was not part of my life plan.

So, I do not practice acupuncture or chiropractic, but there are times when I offer advice. It is a moral obligation to help save a life when you have the knowledge and skill to do it.

One of my first serious cases was an American Taekwondo master who was diagnosed with cancer. I advised him on diet and exercise and he healed completely. Even today, we are still good friends.

One of the managers of a big local company used to come to me for private Taekwondo lessons in the daytime once a week. He had a polyp identified on colonoscopy. I gave him some exercises and advice and by the next visit to the doctor, the polyp had disappeared.

In another case, one of my students had a brother with serious difficulty sleeping and dealing with stress due to marriage and money problems. I had my student pass along a little "homework" for him to do every day. After a week, the brother came in for personal consultation. He had a chronic tightness in his neck and shoulders. I treated him with vigorous massage to the neck, tapping to the head and face, and rubbing around the eyes. Within six months, the brother could sleep and had a new life.

When it comes to therapies like acupuncture, massage and exercise, mental attitude is very important. You must trust the therapy. If it doesn't work, that's okay, but trust it while you try. Skepticism and negative attitudes can ruin even the most effective therapies.

A 7-year-old boy was taking lessons with his family and mother. Both of the parents were chiropractors in the nearby town of Lowell. The boy had a tic with sudden grimaces. This is a sign of a neck problem. I showed the mother what to do to treat the son. There was some abnormality in the 3rd and 4th cervical vertebrae of the neck. She gave a vigorous massage to the neck, tapping to the head and face, and pressure massage around the eyes three to seven times a week. The tic disappeared.

Very simple practices are very effective against even the most difficult medical conditions. Usually they are completely safe as well and have no dangerous side effects. I will share some of these later in the book.

But first, let me tell you about my Life Plan.

Chapter 2 – My Life Plan

Taekwondo... is the way of life

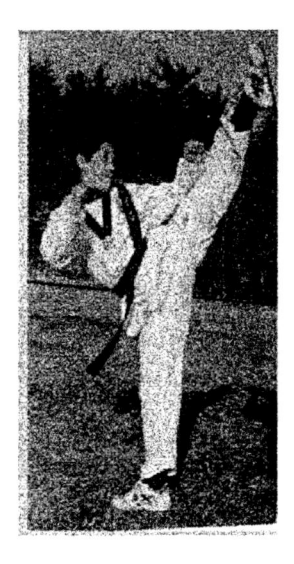

FIVE CODES OF TAEKWONDO
Keep the spirit of Taekwondo
Humility
Integrity
Concentration
Justice

SPIRIT OF TAEKWONDO
Help each other
Respect each other
Self-Control
Self-Discipline
Perseverance

DO JANG RULES
Obey Master
Respect each other
Practice seriously
Keep dojang (TKD school) dean
Keep dobok (uniform) clean
Honest and trustworthy
No smoking
No drinking

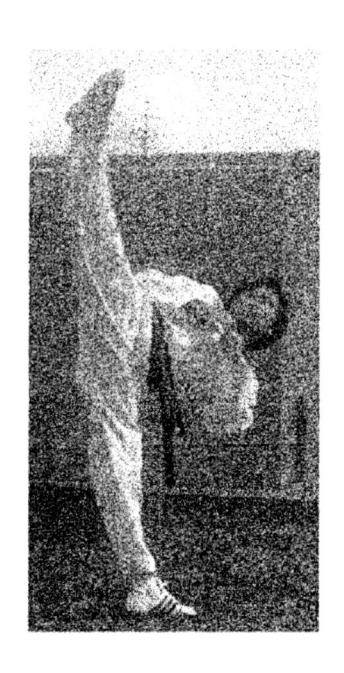

"Taekwondo has given me and my family so much in our lives. Because of training I am able to have a balance of mind, flexibility, disciplined life on food habits and most importantly de-stressing all the stress which is accumulated every day in the life while handling various things. I am growing spiritually more by looking into inner self through Taekwondo. It has also given me an opportunity to know my hidden strengths and skills."

~ Kamala
Brown Belt

"I cannot count the number of times I heard, "Never give up!" Anyone who has spent any time with Grandmaster Kwon will know that "never give up" relates to everything in your life. Grandmaster Kwon inspires us all to keep trying to be better. Not only better at Taekwondo, but better instructors, students, friends, parents, children...basically, better people."

~ Master David Esposito
6th Dan Black Belt
Esposito family / Southern Maine TKD

May 8, 1987 marks my new birth in America. I was not yet even 40 but knew what I would devote my life to – Taekwondo!

Taekwondo is more than just a martial art. It is the national sport of Korea, like baseball or football here, and is practiced everywhere – at home, in the parks, at schools and universities and, of course, in the military. It is a fitness system with a philosophy that applies to all life and society. (I like to think of our school as a martial arts-based family fitness system.)

In 1987, I wrote up my life plan. Everyone should have a life plan to guide them and correct them when they stray. Otherwise, how will you know how you are doing? Here are the nine points that guide my life:

1. Be humble.

2. My Taekwondo uniform is my life and my best friend.

3. My blood and sweat are the seeds of my life.

4. Laziness is my worst enemy.

5. Show action, not just words.

6. Life is a marathon.

7. Never give up.

8. Take responsibility.

9. Life doesn't come to you, you must go after it.

These simple words are worth thinking about. I meditate on them every day. You must choose your own plan and your own words, but these are mine.

Be humble. Humility is one of the Five Codes of Taekwondo. It means to live and behave modestly. I think of this whenever I'm tempted to show off.

My Taekwondo uniform is my life and my best friend. I still have the *dobok* (uniform) and black belt I brought with me from Korea in 1987. It reminds me of my commitment to excellence in this discipline.

My blood and sweat are the seeds of my life. All things worthwhile in life come through hard work. If you don't work for something, you won't value it. Hard work is both the way to success and the key to enjoying it.

Laziness is my worst enemy. Being lazy will stop any plan from fulfillment. The time to start anything is now. Keep going and never give up!

Show action, not just words. Taekwondo is about action, not talk. Whether it is fitness, health, education, work, or relationships, words must be put into motion. Things don't get done by themselves. Don't tell yourself to do something 100 times. Write it down and do it.

Life is a marathon. Everything worthwhile takes time. Don't be impatient, just keep going.

Never give up. Perseverance is the greatest of virtues and part of the Spirit of Taekwondo. Most people fail because they stop trying.

Take responsibility. Never be afraid to say, "I'm sorry," even when it isn't your fault. Don't let your pride and arrogance escalate arguments into fighting and rage.

Life doesn't come to you, you must go after it. You must reach out and grasp what life offers. Seek out what you want and pursue it with all your might!

"(The) level of skill (of Grandmaster Kwon) is like nothing I had ever seen – in real life or in the movies. He is insanely flexible, quick, and masterful. He is wise, approachable, and kind. He exudes such strength – of body, mind, and character!

One day as I was watching a class, a young boy about 7 years old started to cry. He couldn't do the move that was being asked of him. In utter frustration, he started to leave the dojang.

"Focus. Just try to do your best," said Grandmaster Kwon, and he put his hand on the young boy's shoulder. "That's all you have to do, is try to do your best." The boy looked up at Grandmaster Kwon's face, and from where I sat, a calmness and strength passed from the grandmaster to the young boy. The boy resisted running from the studio, and he tried again. He squashed his internal battle between fear and frustration. With the Grandmaster as his guide, the young boy stayed to practice and fought against his urge to give up."

~ Dana Yerid
Brown-White Belt

Chapter 3 – Daily Habits That Lead to Health

"I like to bob up and down on the balls of my feet, as that helps me to quickly wake up in the morning and overcome the mental malaise that sets in when my circadian rhythm dips each afternoon. Another thing I find very helpful is self-massage. Grandmaster Kwon has shown me how to combine hand-tapping and break-falling to not only overcome back spasms but reunite all parts of the body. It's interesting, how the entire body tingles with energy after this exercise; but I am most grateful because it has helped me overcome pain and greatly improve my range-of-motion."

~ Mark Fortune
3rd Dan Black Belt

I have a few practical habits to share with you that will help you stay fit and healthy long into old age. They are simple and very basic. They are not hard to do, do not take much time, and are very effective.

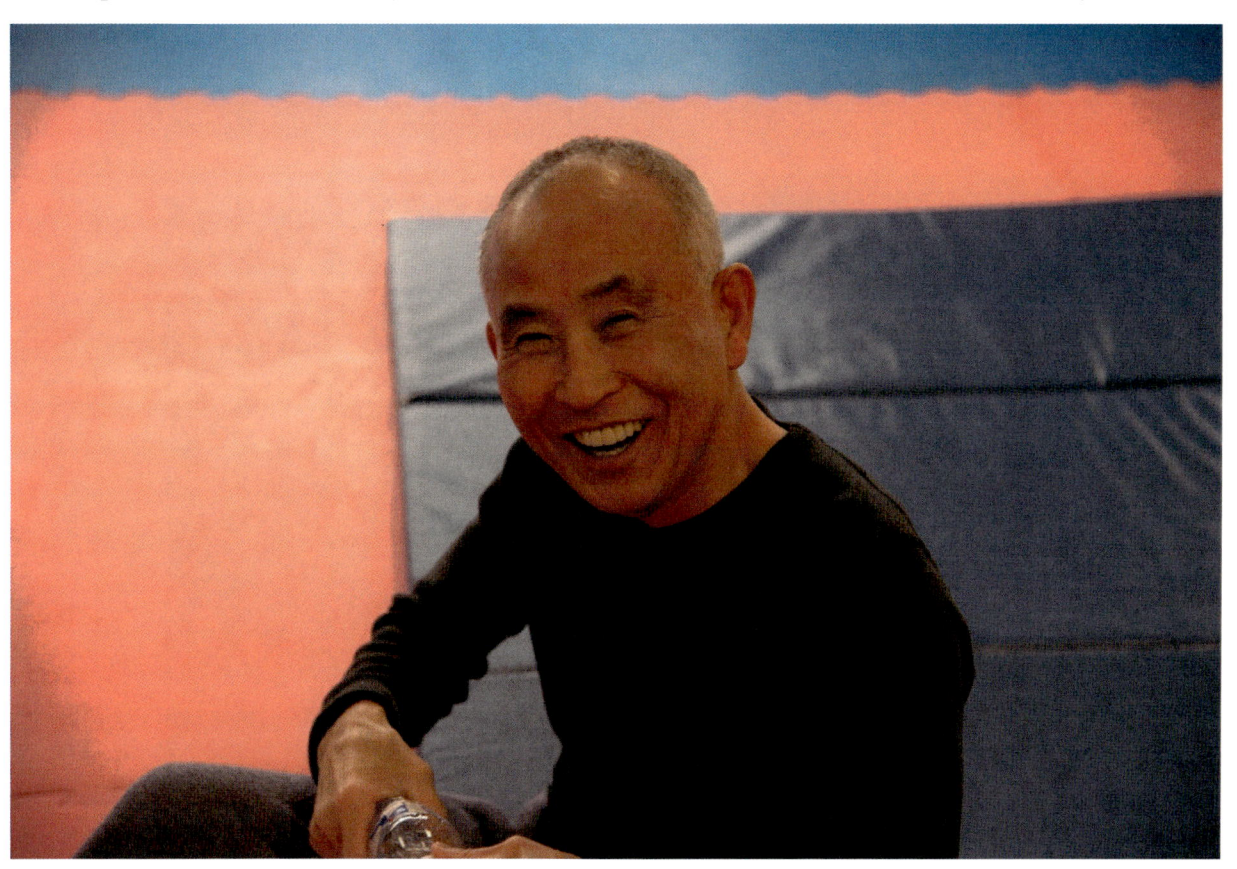

Getting out of bed

Before rising, spend a few minutes moving all your joints, starting with your feet and ankles – flex, extend, rotate.

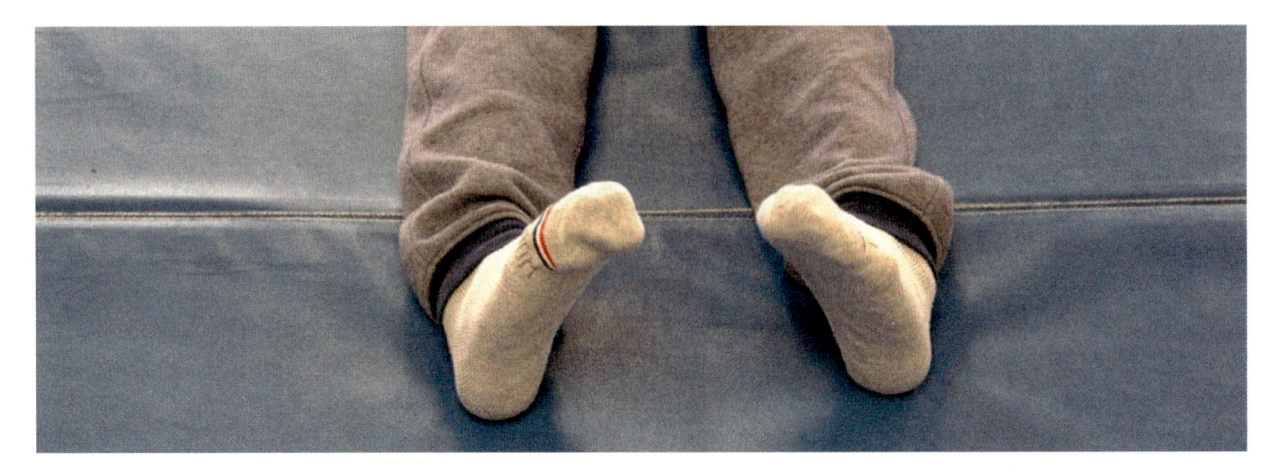

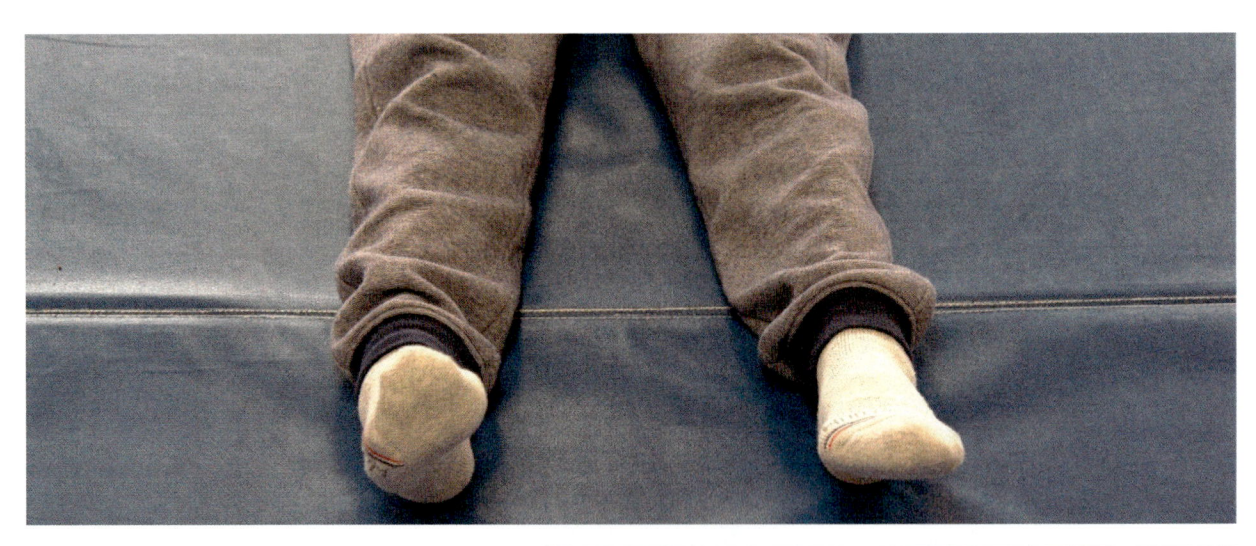

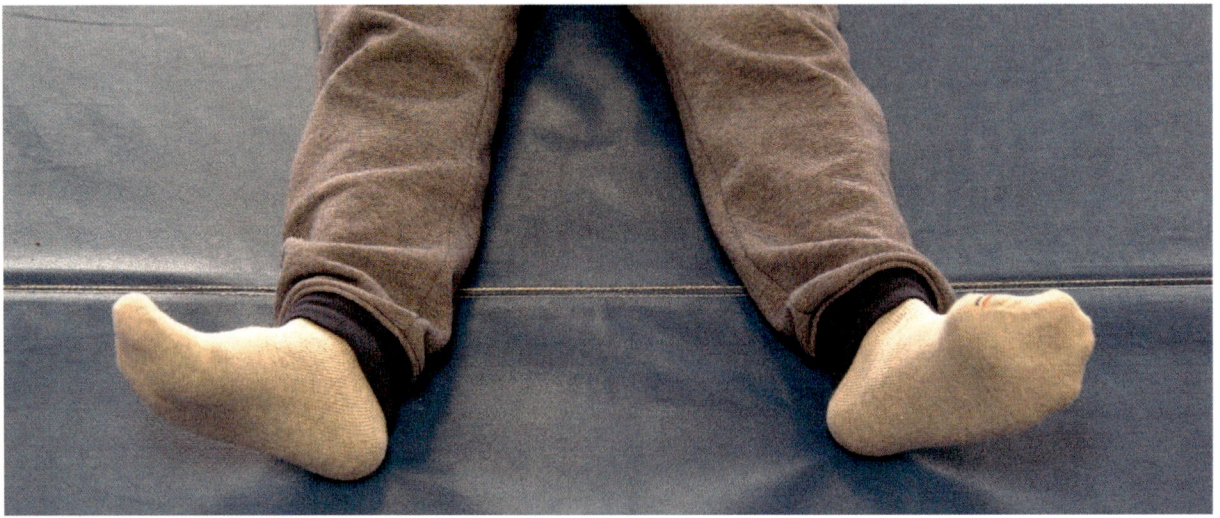

Then bend the knees and bicycle slowly, stretching them out and up.

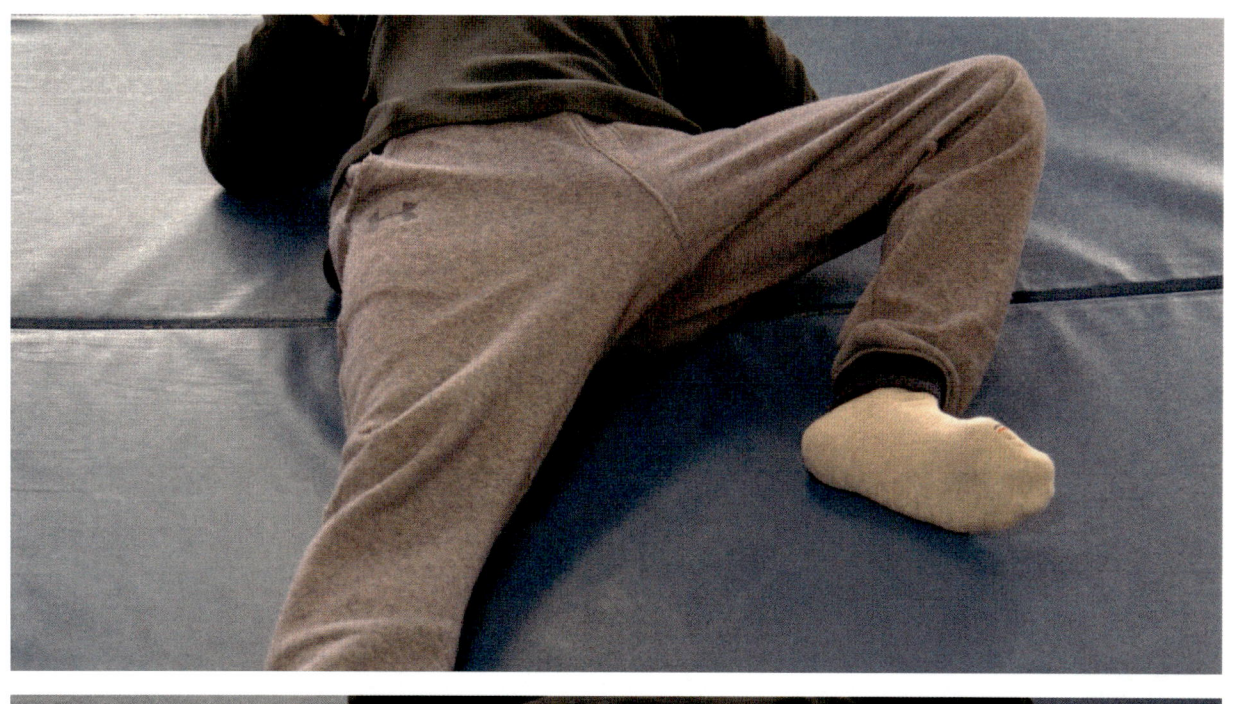

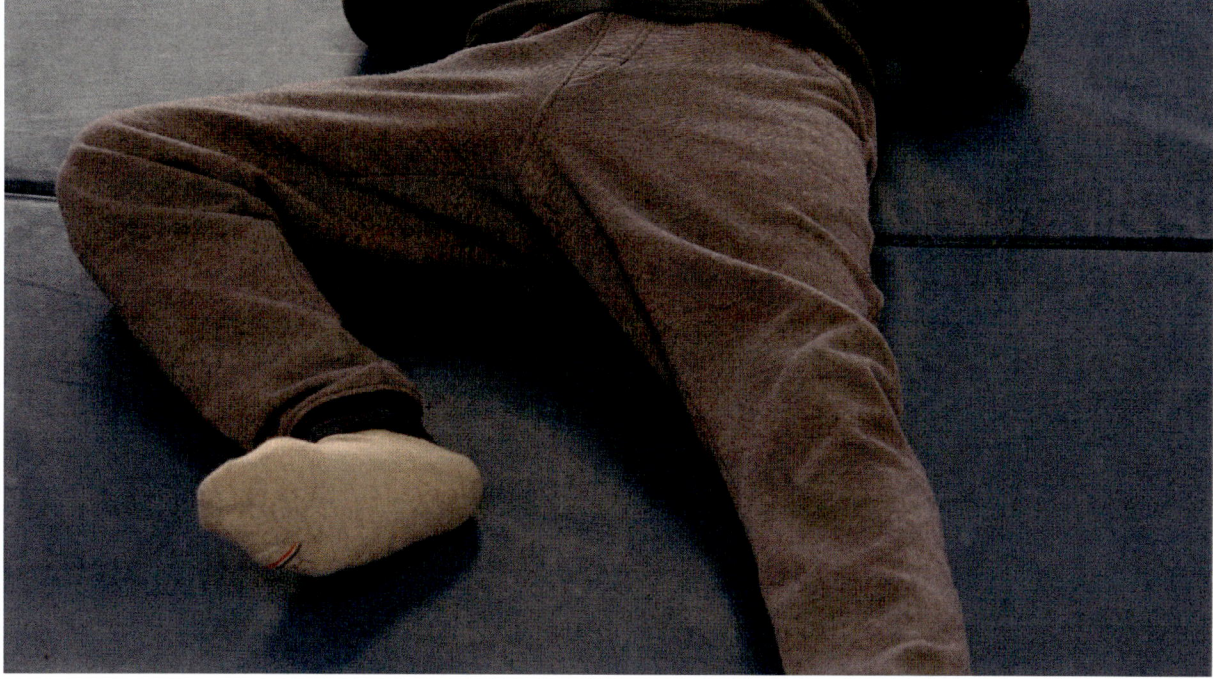

Twist at the waist, bending from one side to the other.

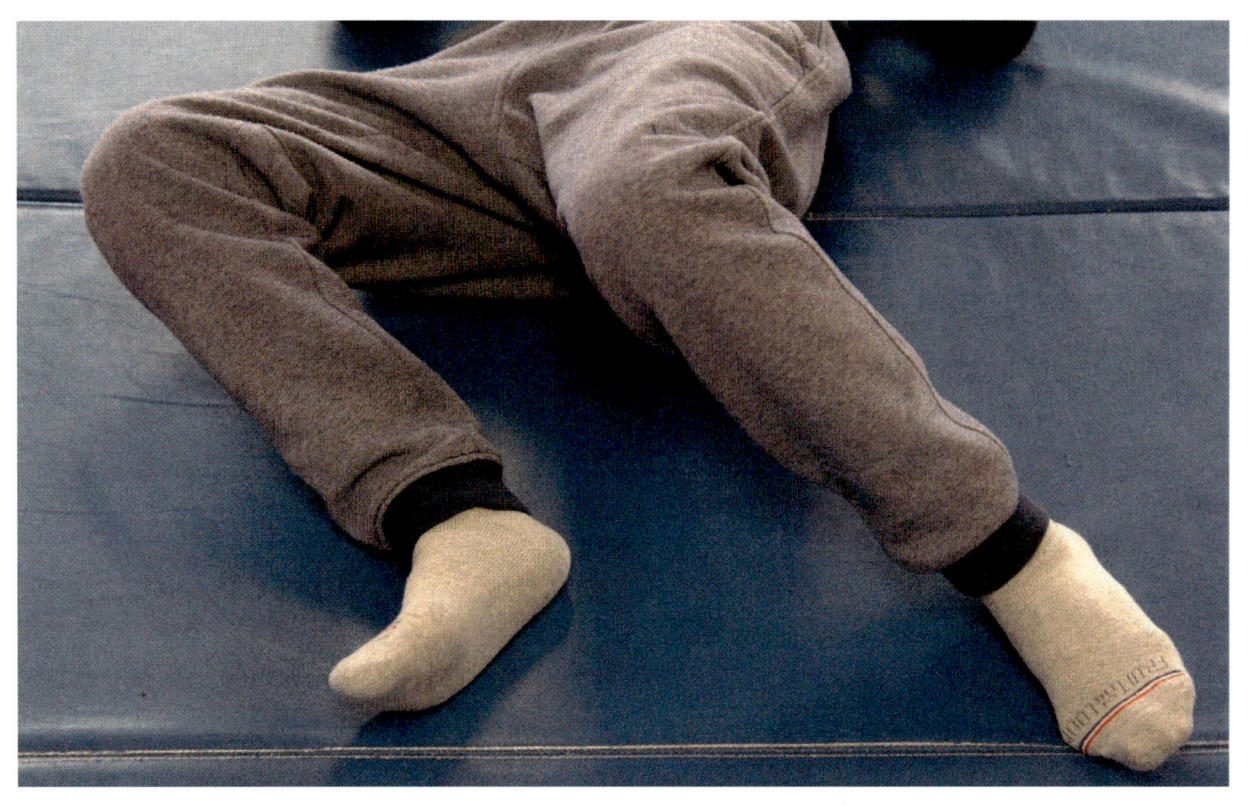

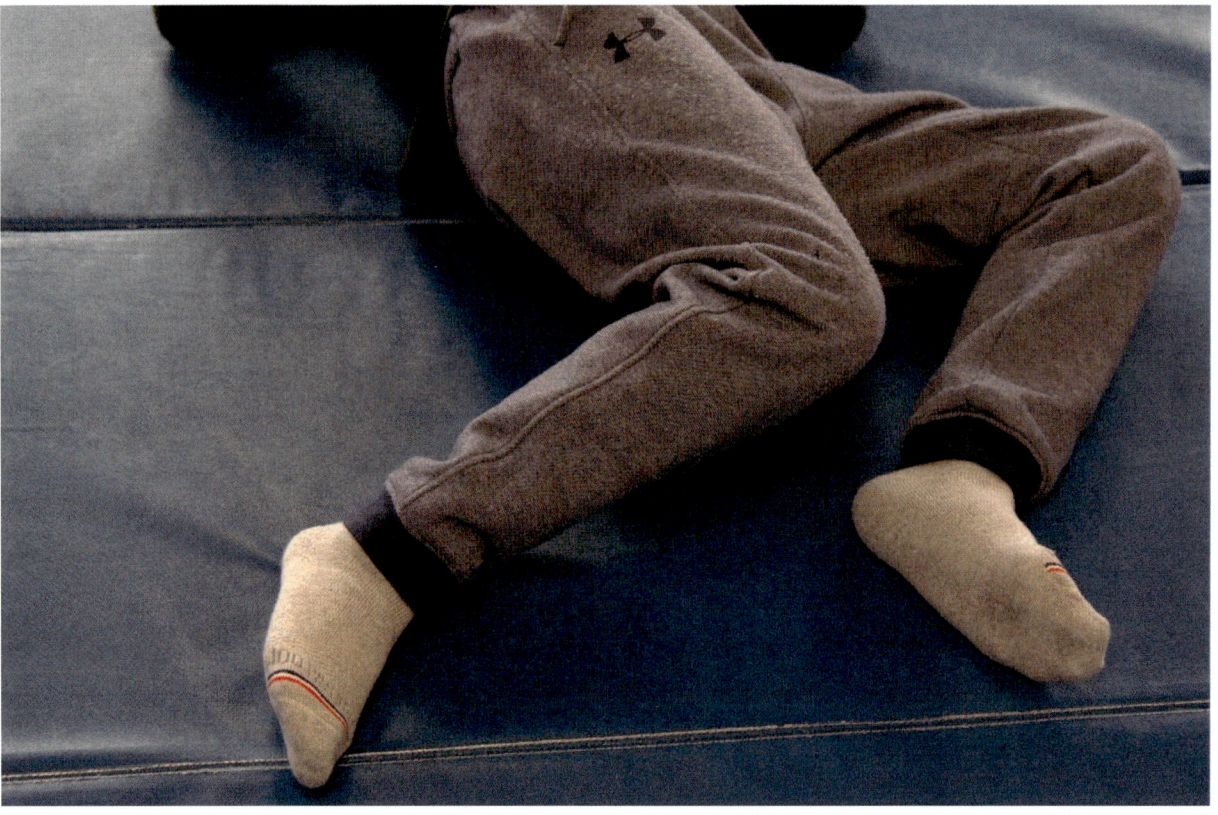

Roll the whole body from side to side a few times.

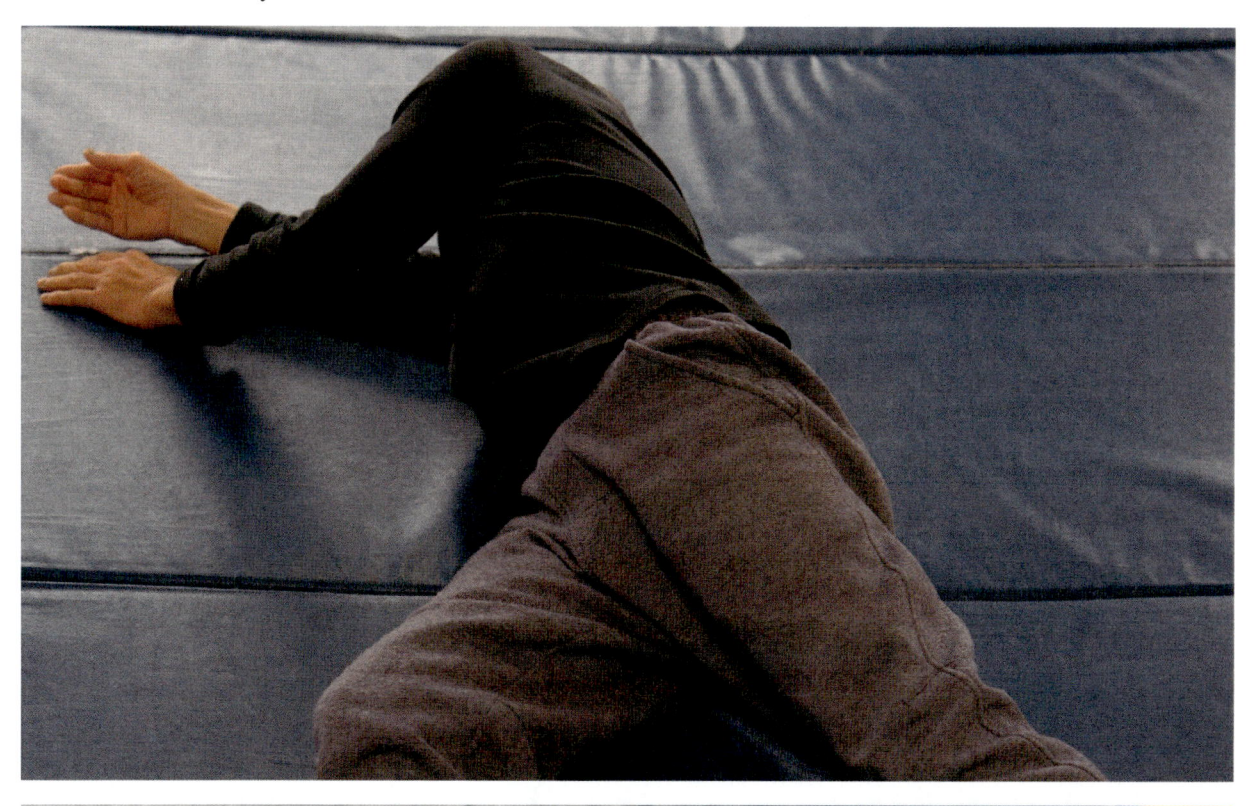

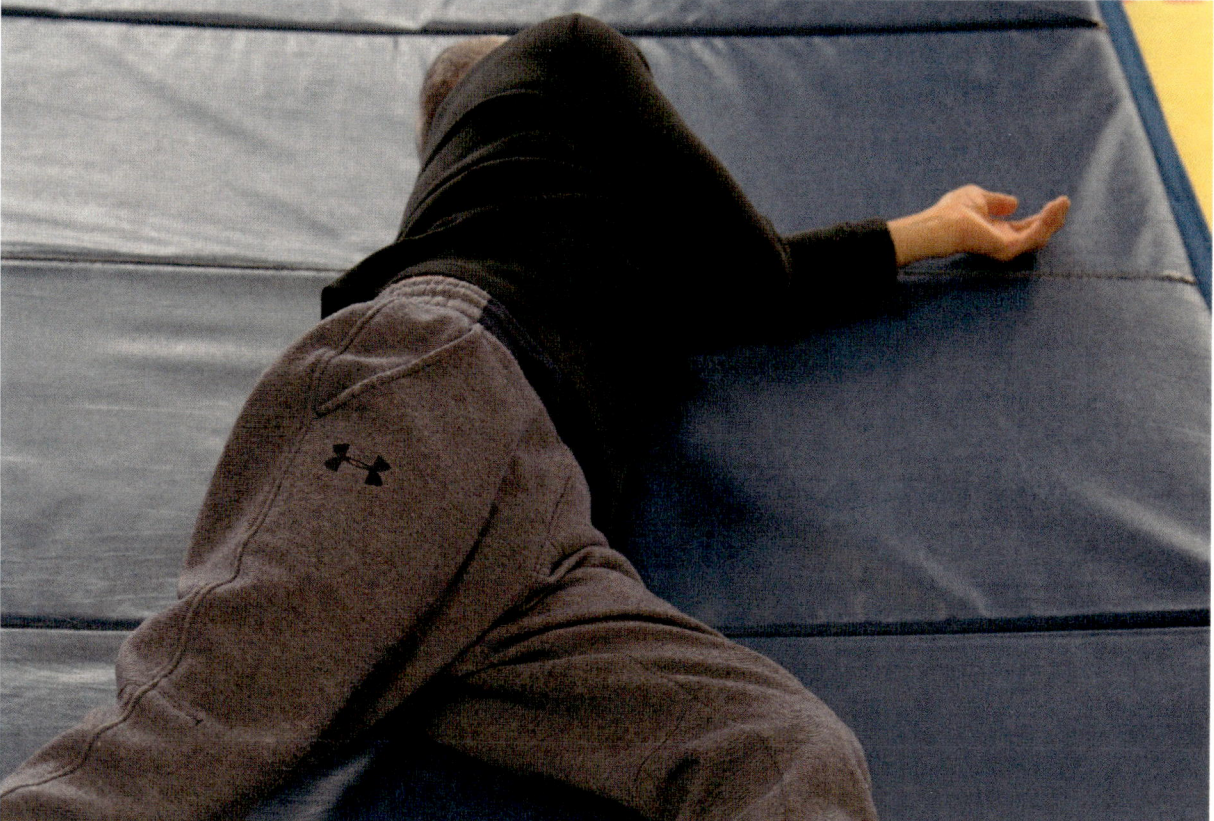

Lying flat on your back in bed, stretch your arms straight up.

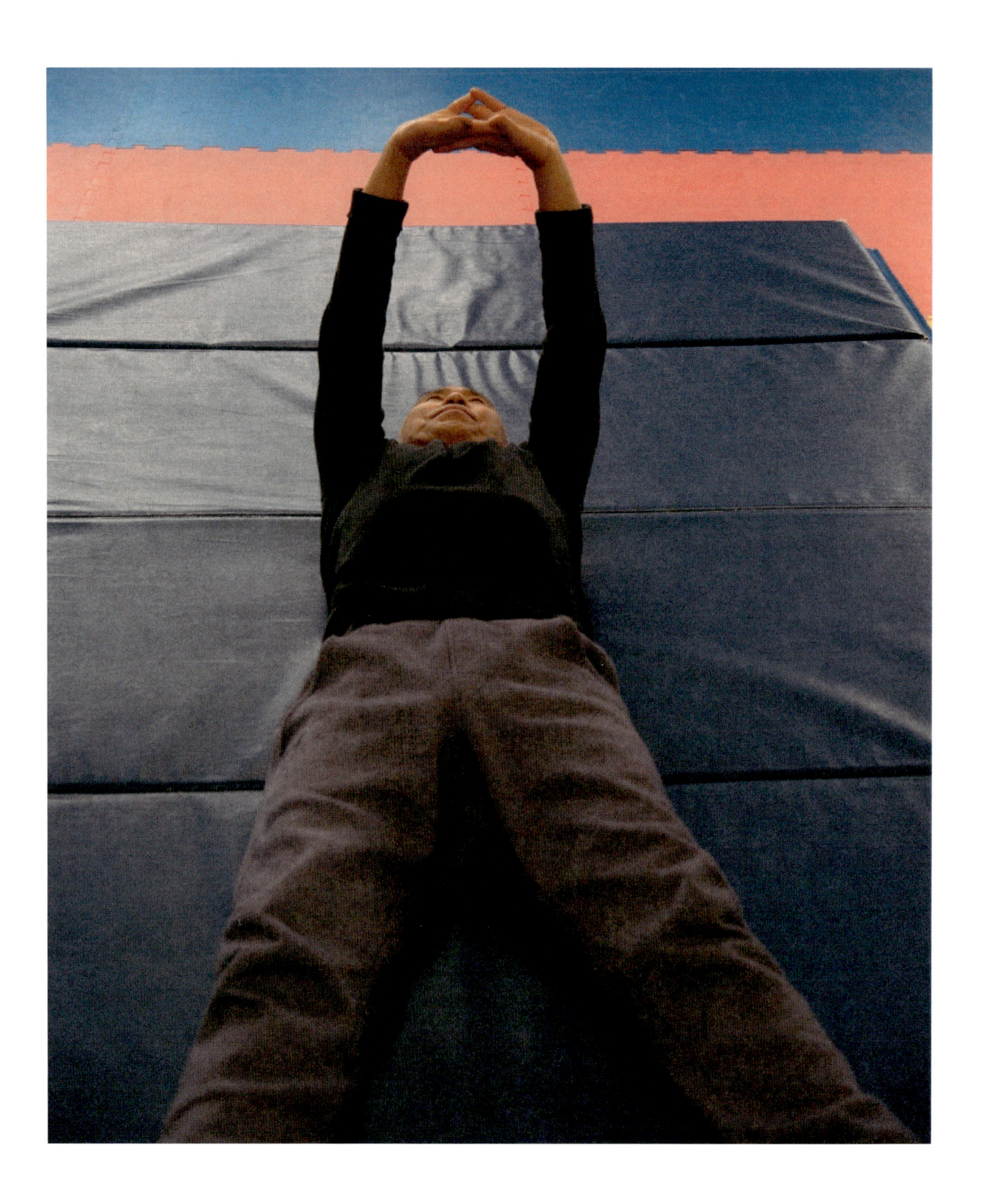

Rotate your shoulders in all directions a few times.

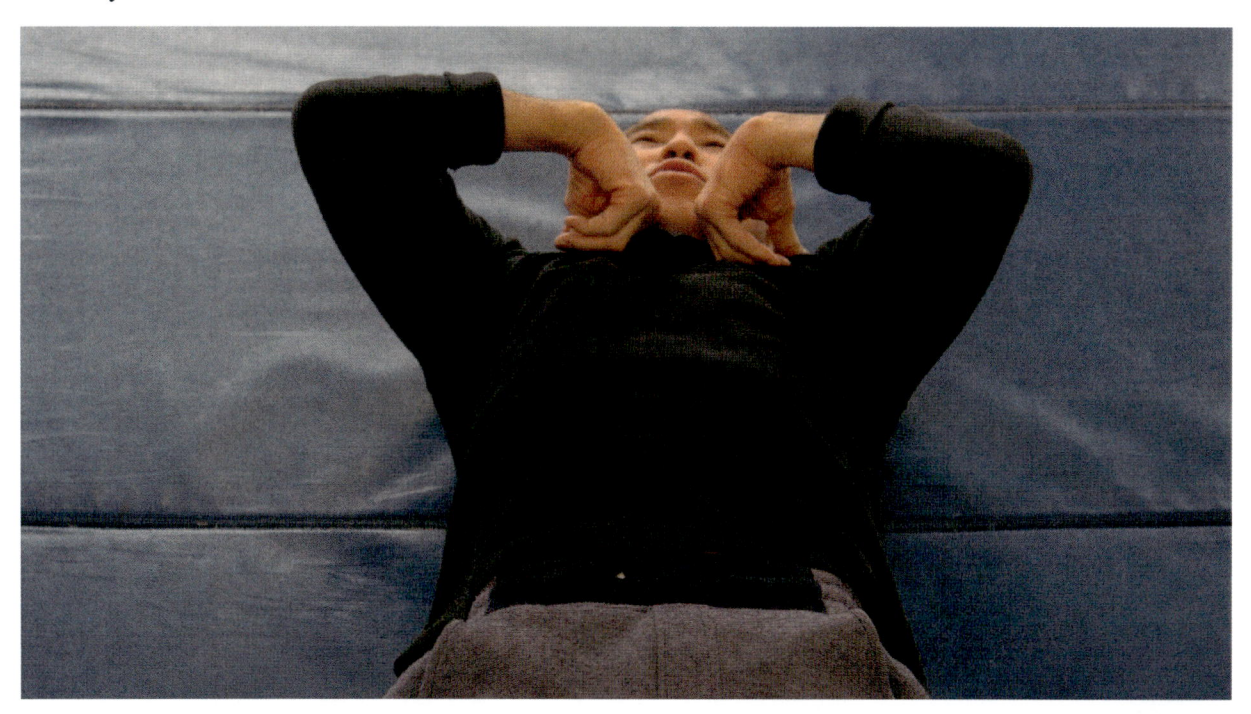

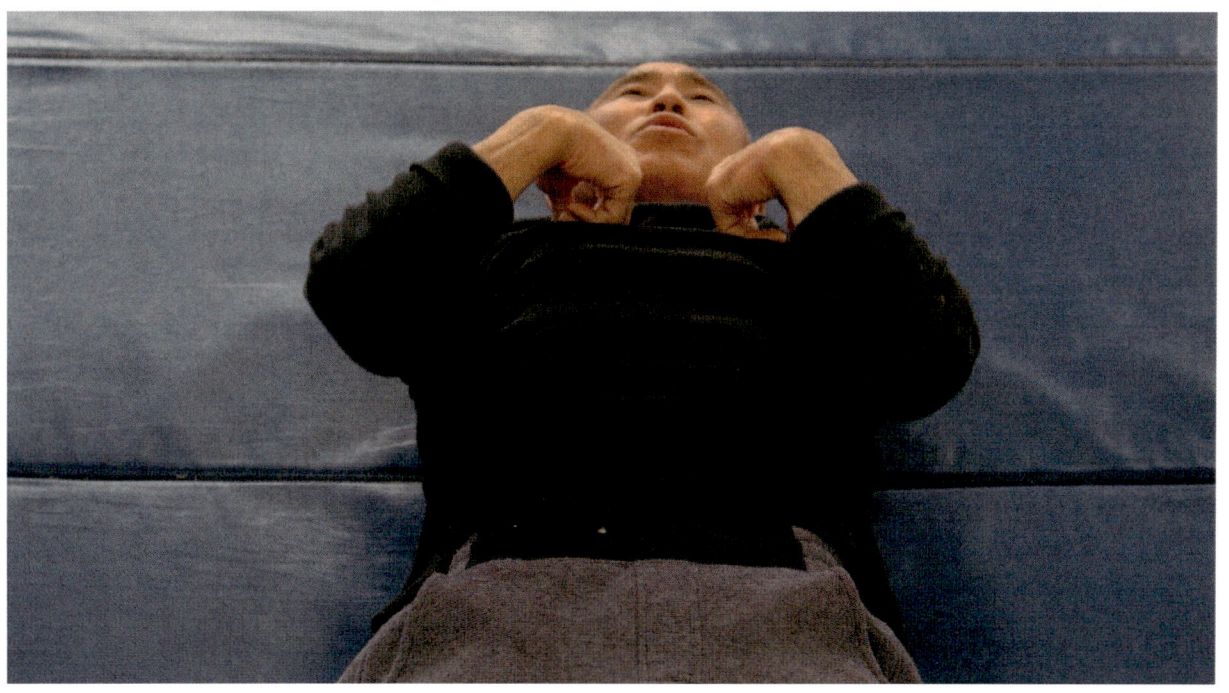

Still lying on your back, take a deep breath into the belly and tighten your stomach muscles and pelvic floor.

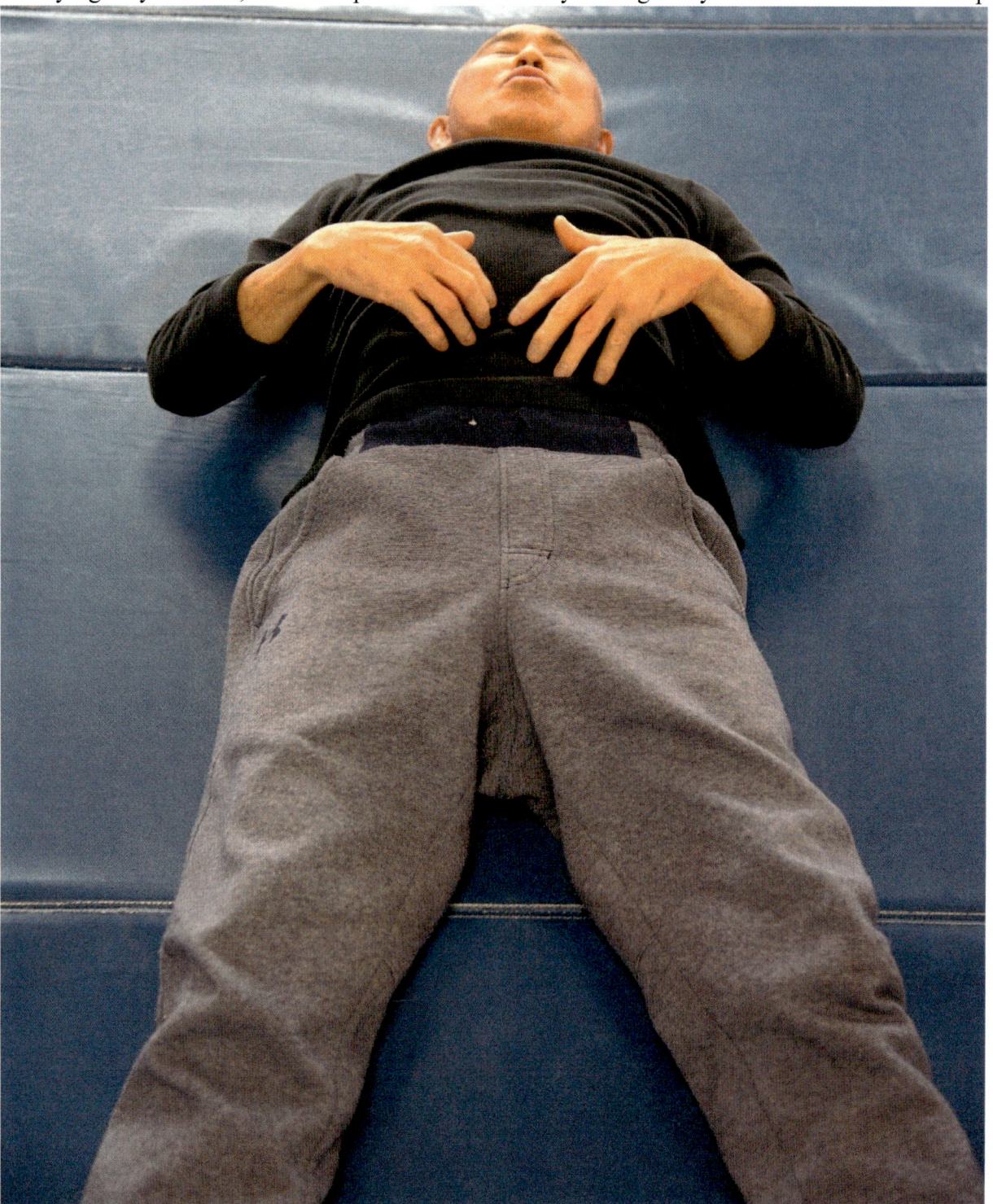

Do small crunches with hands on the belly while holding your breath. Do maybe 20 to 30 quick repetitions. Don't bend the neck.

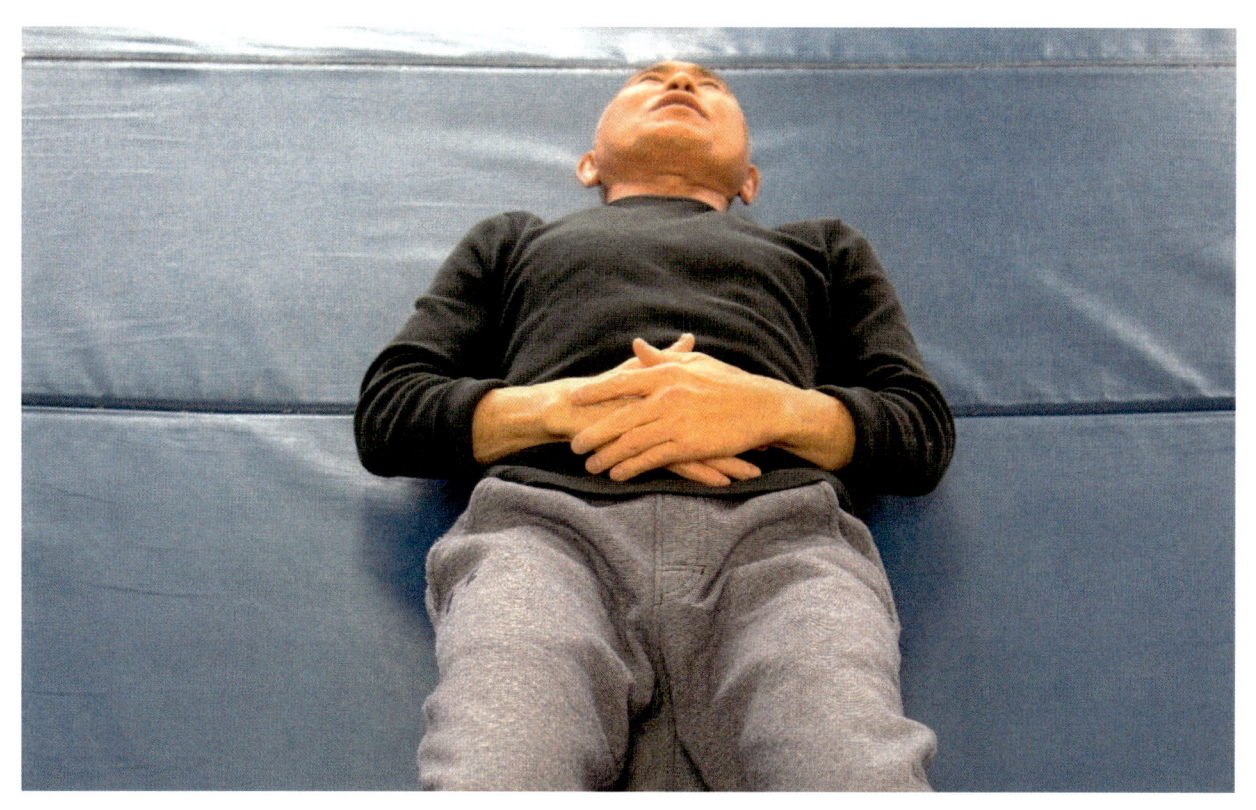

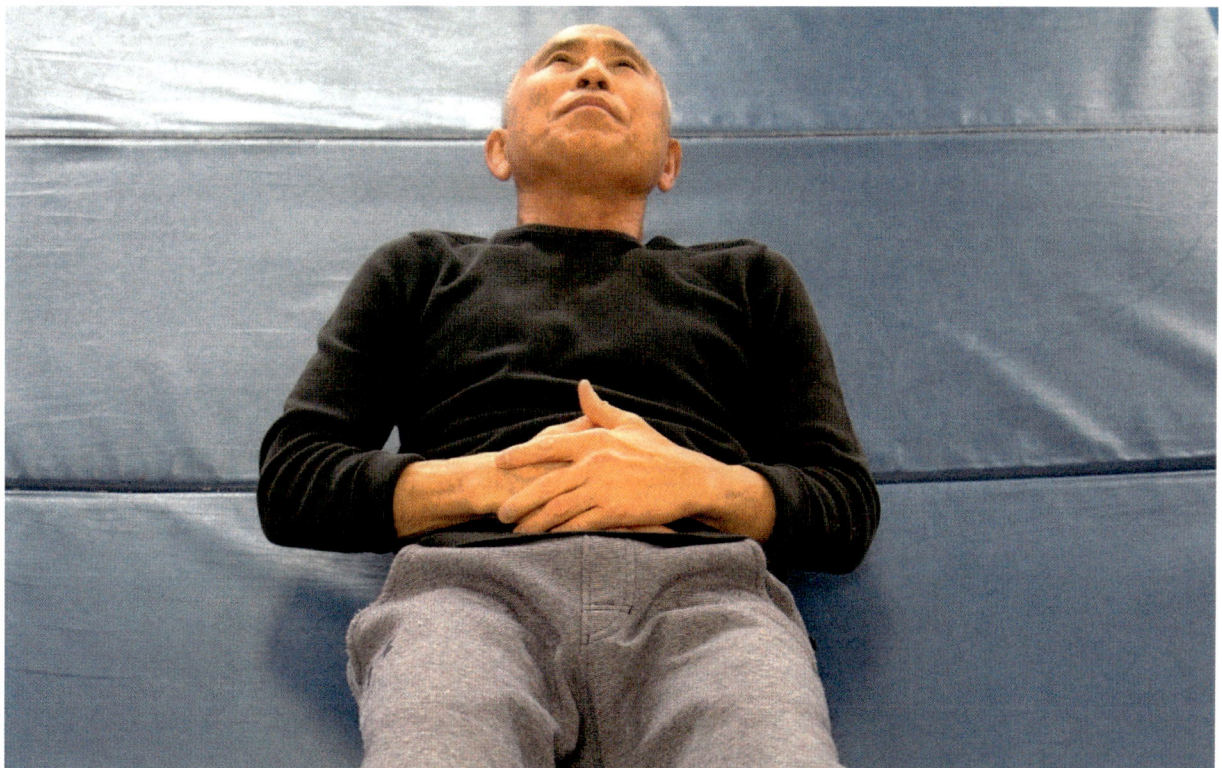

Now you can get out of bed.

Starting the Day

While in the bathroom, stand on your toes or do calf raises while shaving and brushing your teeth.

In the shower, squat down low and let the water hit you with force. It's a water massage for your head and shoulders. Tap and slap yourself all over. The shower is the best time for self-massage and warm up exercise. Include a calf stretch if you have room. End the shower with cold water to tighten and tone up the skin. It will really wake you up!

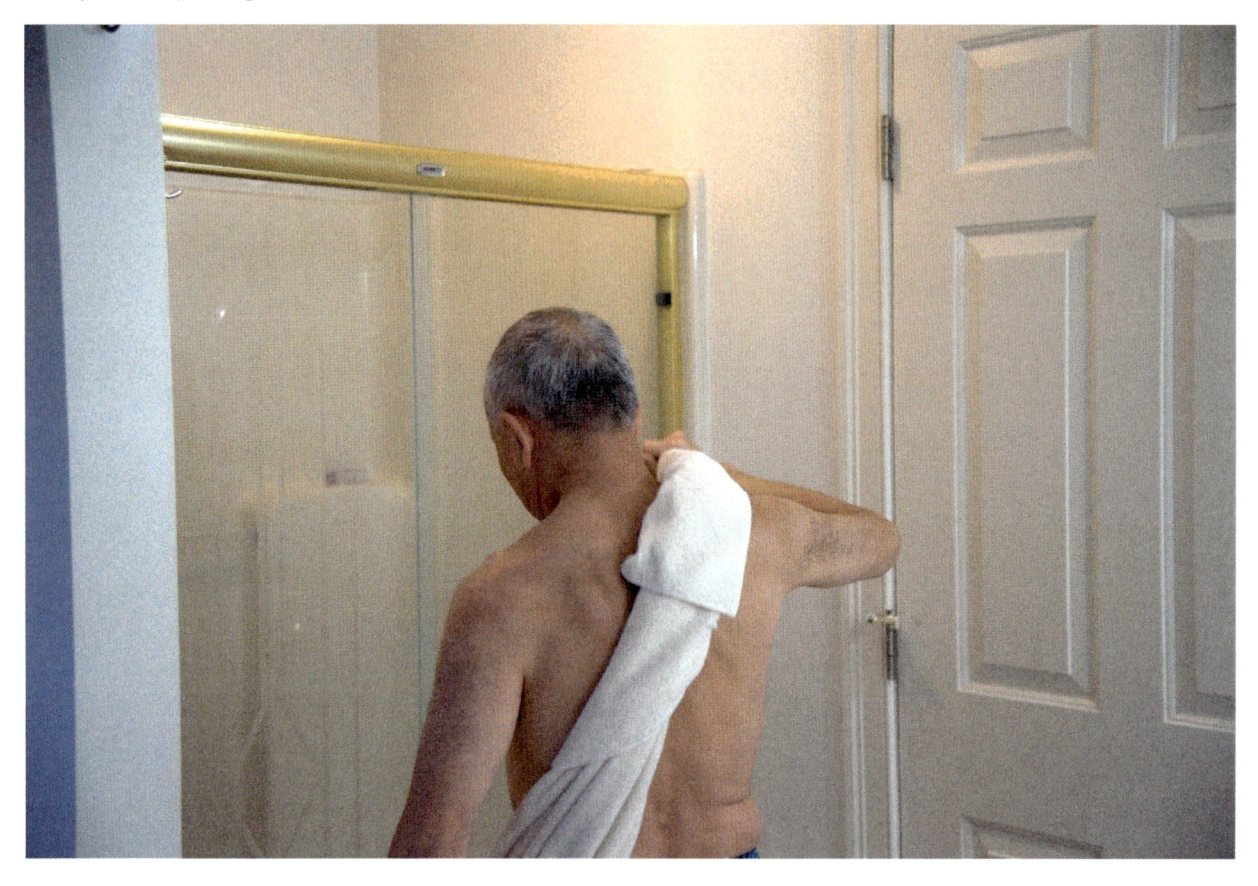

Towel off with a rough towel to make the skin happy and move your arms and shoulders. Massage with tapping, slapping, and bumping is better than lotion to give your skin a healthy pink glow. Sending the vibrations deep into the internal organs is very good for them as well and helps the internal circulation. It keeps the good energy flowing freely.

After all this, you will have tapped, slapped, and massaged every inch of your body except your back. So, find a place to lie down, perhaps on a piece of carpet or yoga mat. Lie on your back with your knees bent. Lift up your hips and gently bump the sacrum on floor a few times.

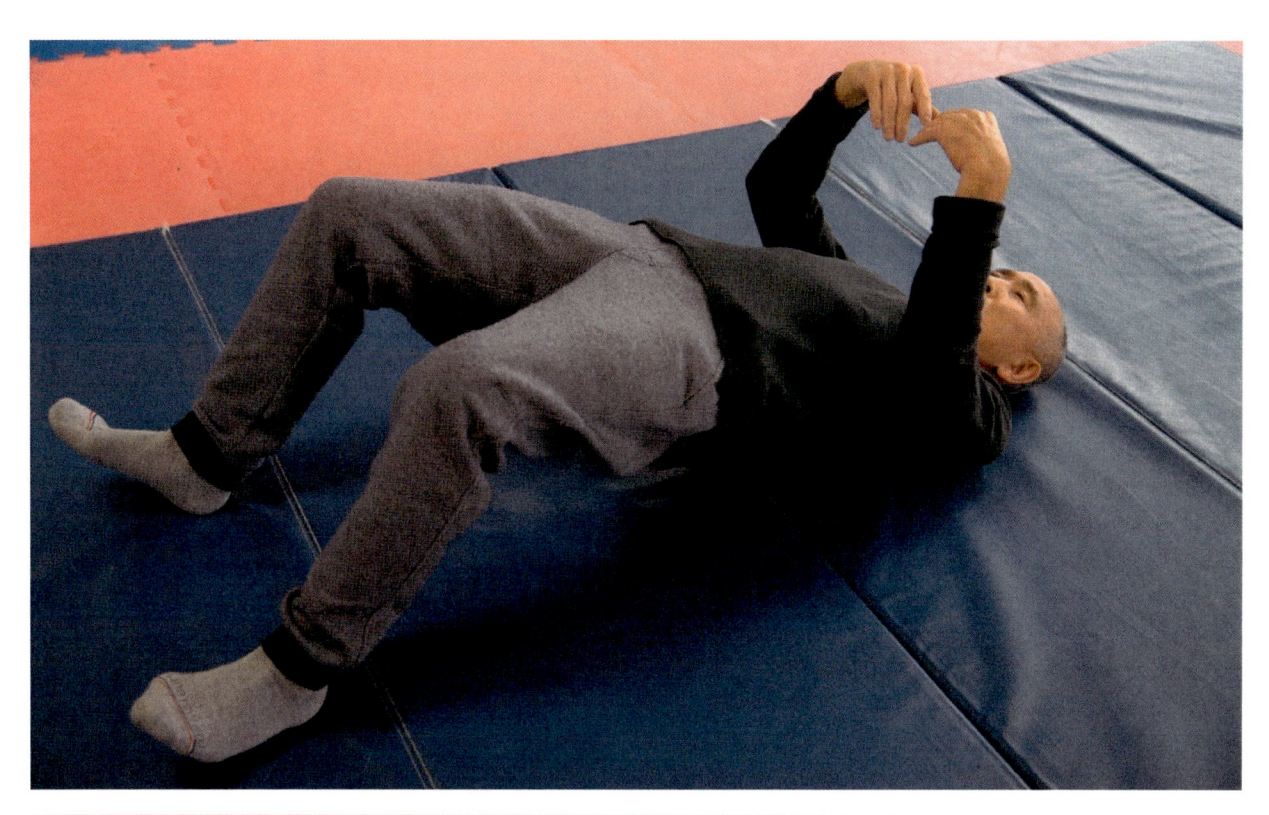

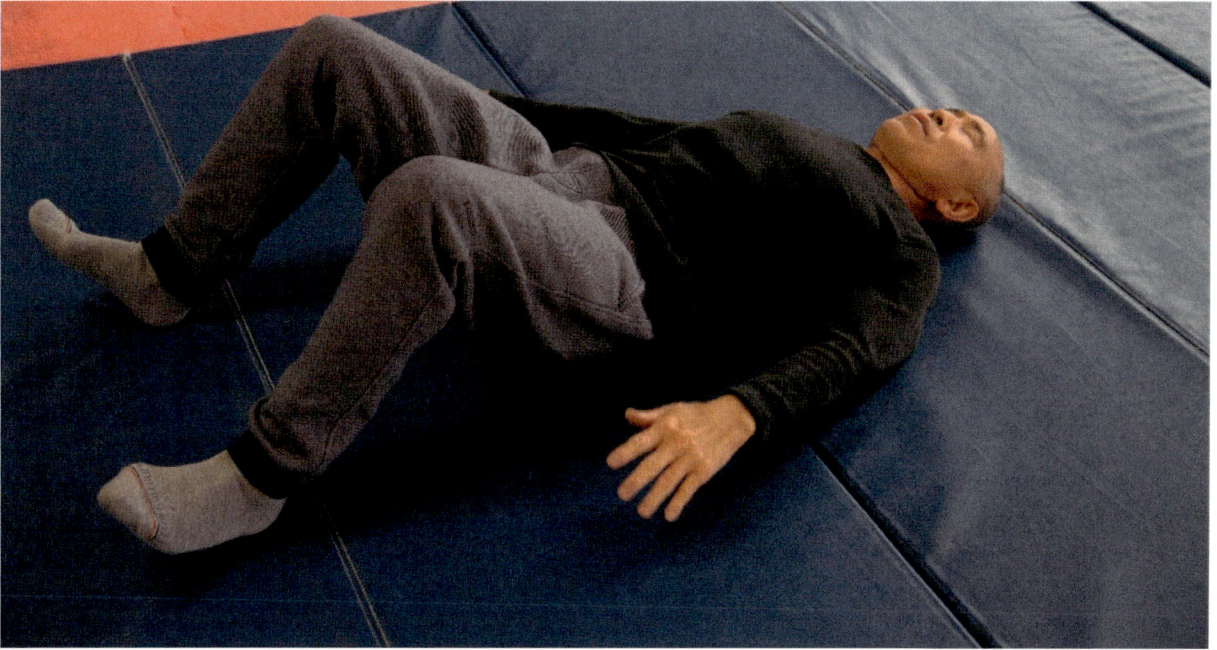

Governing Vessel

The governing vessel[2] of the body that runs up and down the middle of the body is very important. We pay attention to the front of our bodies, but not so much to the back. All of the universe is a balance of *um* and *yang*. Exercises to stimulate the governing vessel at the back are important to balance the front.

At work and travel

You must get out of the chair and move around at least once every 90 minutes. Two hours at most!

Stretch out all your joints. Twist your spine and bend it in all directions. Work your muscles by doing isometric exercises and lifting yourself in your chair. If you can, stand up and take a few moments to do a low front stance and horseback stance.

If you are driving, find time to pull over and get out to stretch and move. Every 90 minutes! When flying, try to get up and move as often as you can.

Besides getting up and moving around, tapping and beating gently on your head and limbs will stimulate circulation. Circulation is key! Energy that flows freely will keep you young. Tight muscles and stiff joints block the flow of energy.

---

[2] The student of Traditional Chinese Medicine will recognize the concepts of yin (*um* in Korean) and *yang* as well as *qi gong* (*ki gong* in Korean). Throughout the book we will keep the Korean terms.

The governing vessel is the confluence of all the *yang* channels, which it governs. The governing and conception vessels are two branches of the inseparable *um* and *yang*, front-back duality. Regulating the governing and conception vessels is a priority in medical *ki gong*. Along these vessels, the *yang* fire and *um* essence flow up and down the body along these vessels, bringing the water and fire energies together. This fusion creates the *um-yang* balance throughout the body.

"The Conception vessel and the Governing vessel are like midnight and midday, they are the polar axis of the body ... there is one source and two branches, one goes to the front and the other to the back of the body ... When we try to divide these, we see that yin and yang are inseparable. When we try to see them as one, we see that it is an indivisible whole."

~Li Shizhen

[Li Shizhen (Chinese: 李時珍) was a Han Chinese polymath, medical doctor, scientist, pharmacologist, herbalist and acupuncturist of the Ming dynasty. His major contribution to clinical medicine was his 27-year work, which is found in his scientific book *Compendium of Materia Medica*. He is also considered to be the greatest scientific naturalist of China. (https://en.wikipedia.org/wiki/Li_Shizhen)]

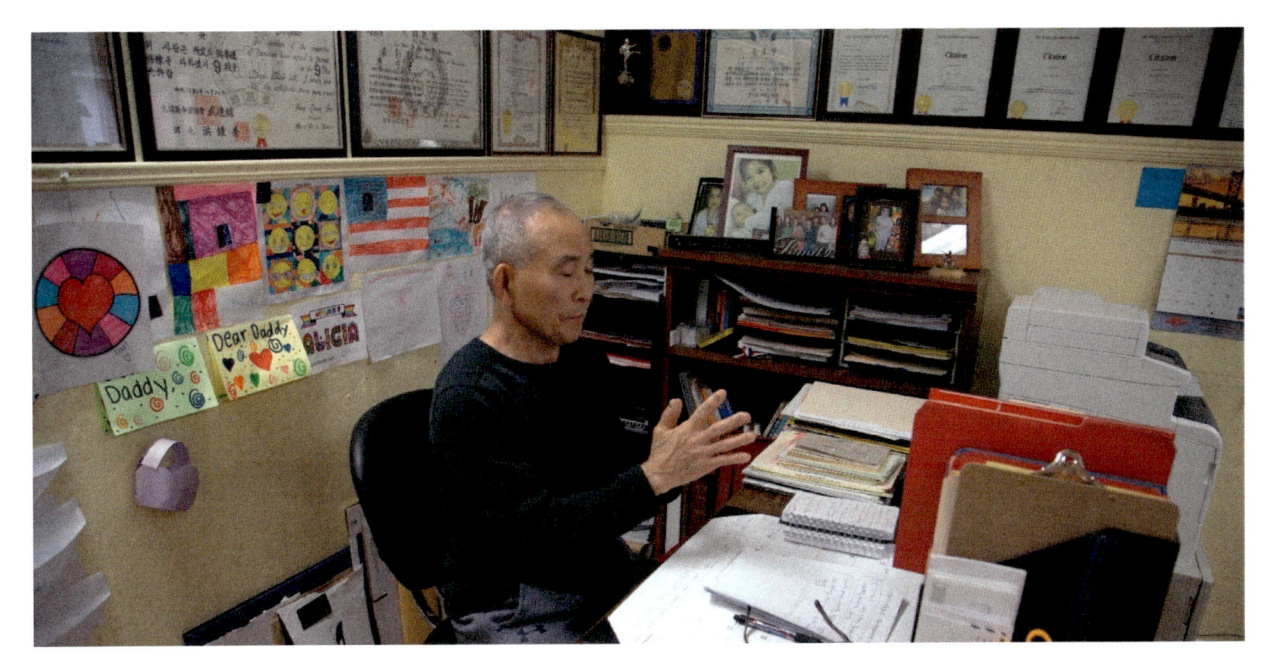

If you work at a desk job, you see the effects that sitting in a hunched over posture can have over the years. Your body eventually molds itself into a bent and stiff posture.

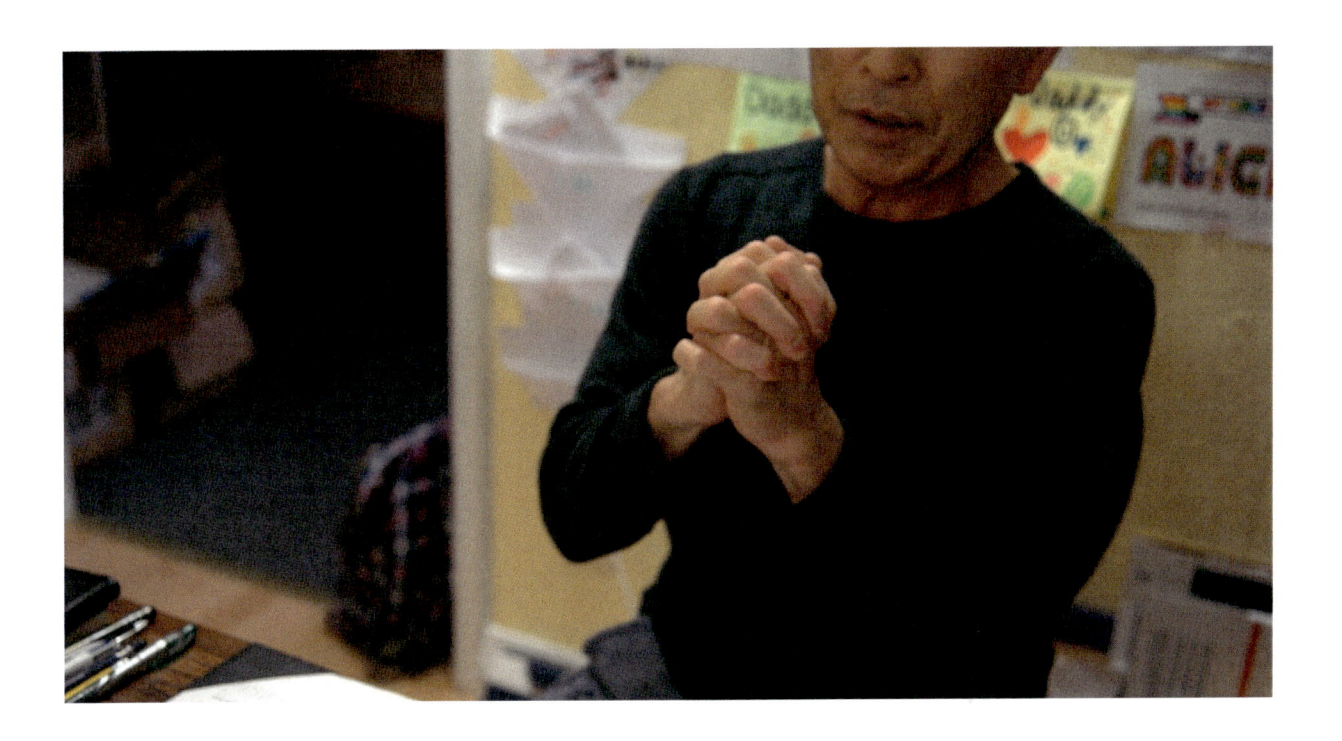

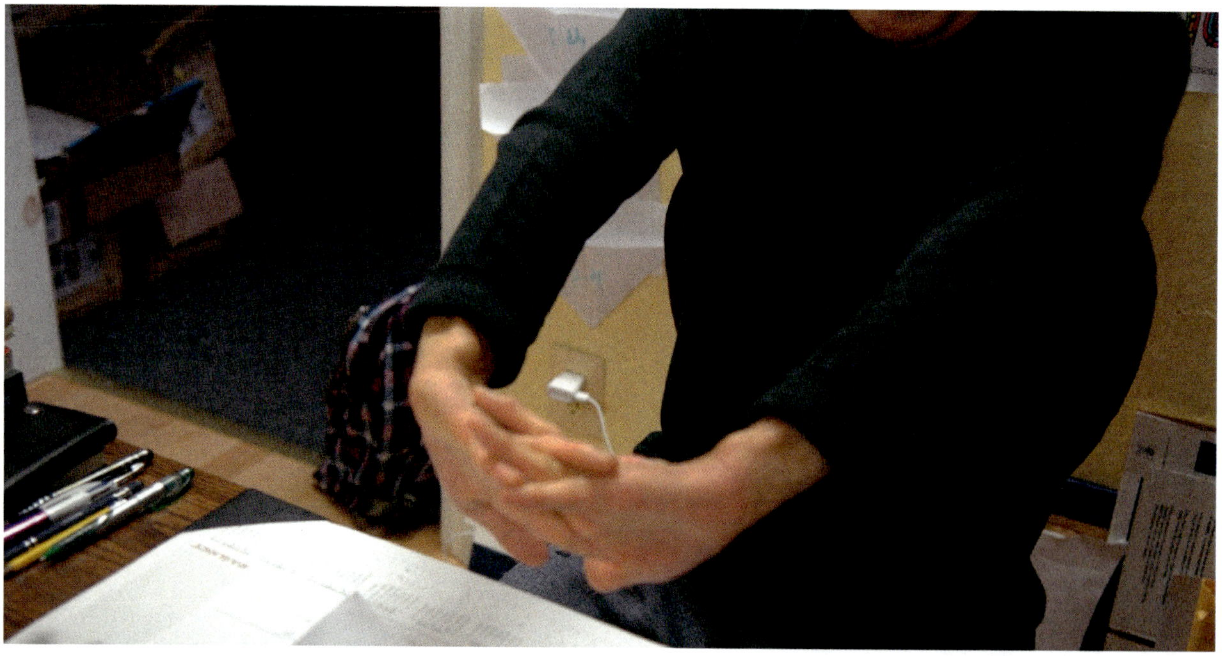

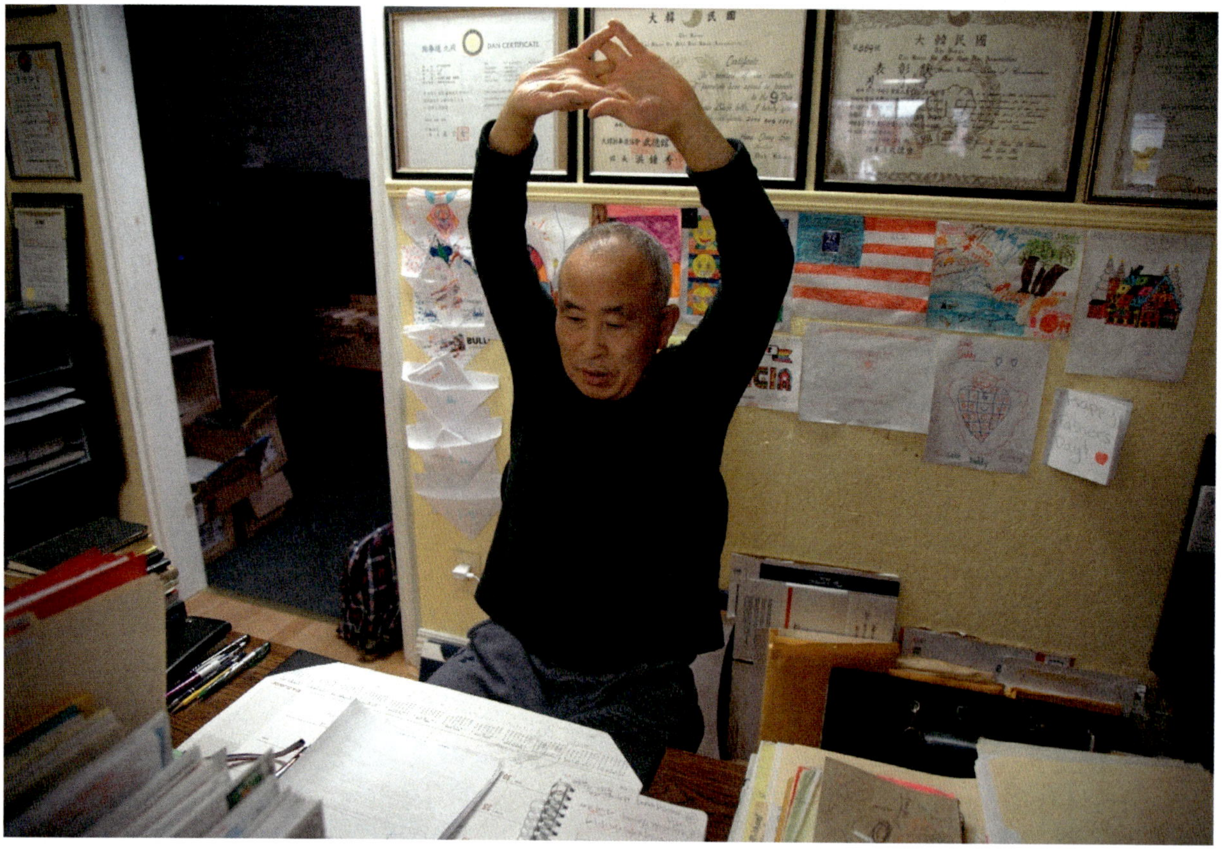

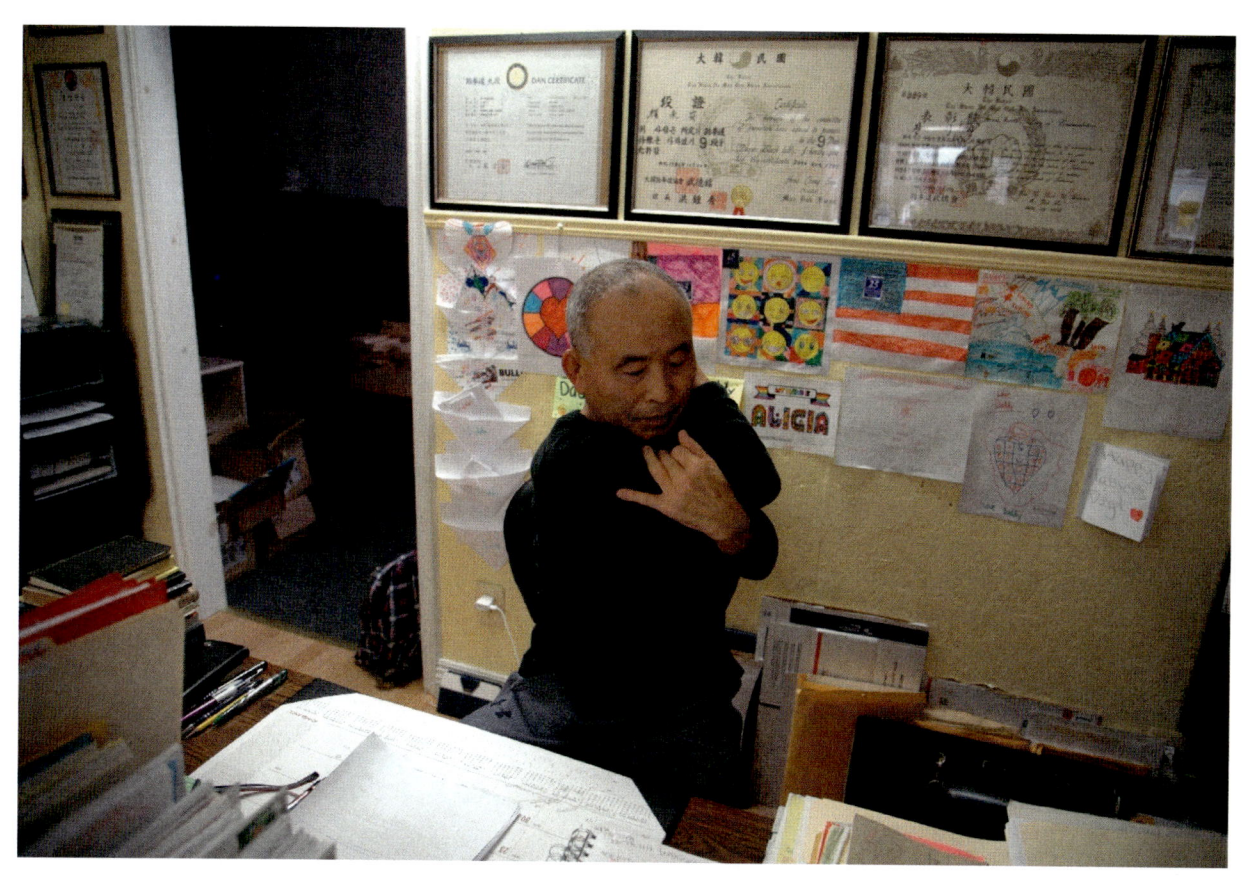

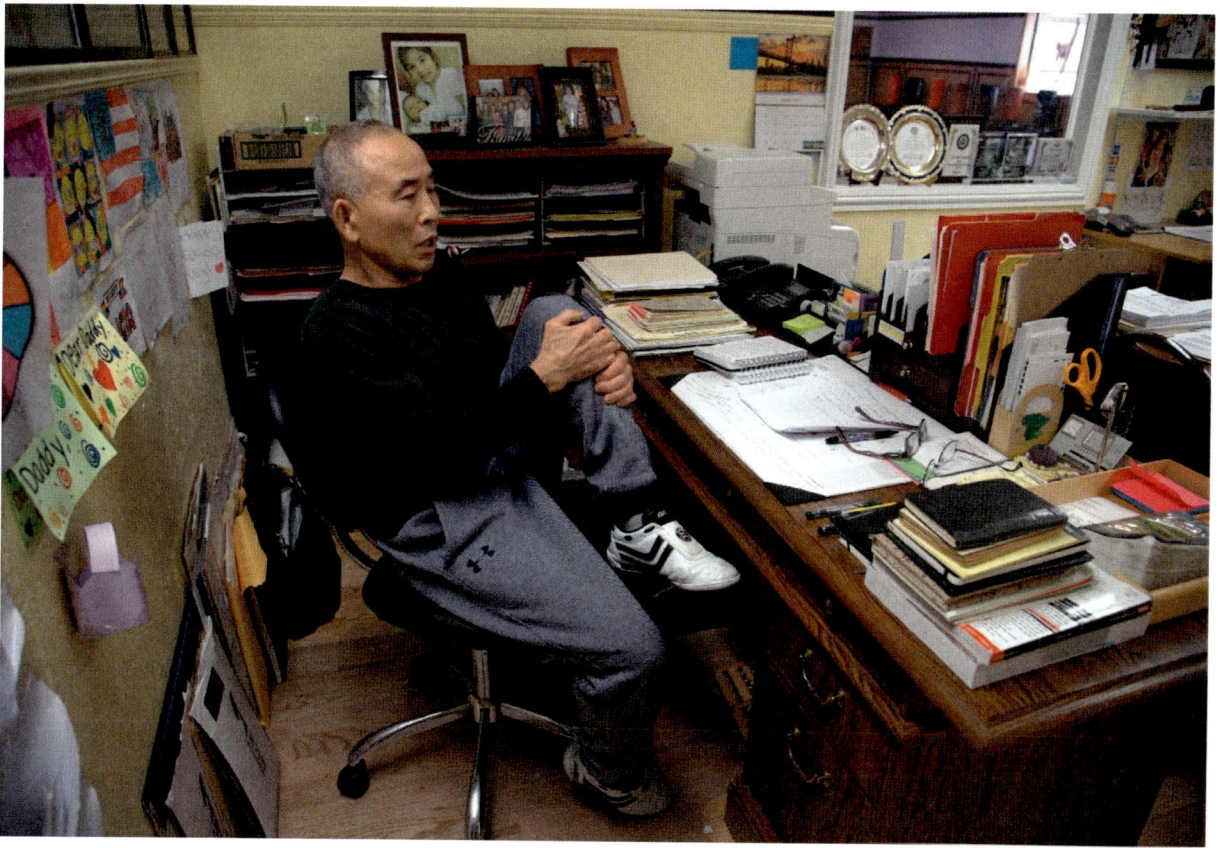

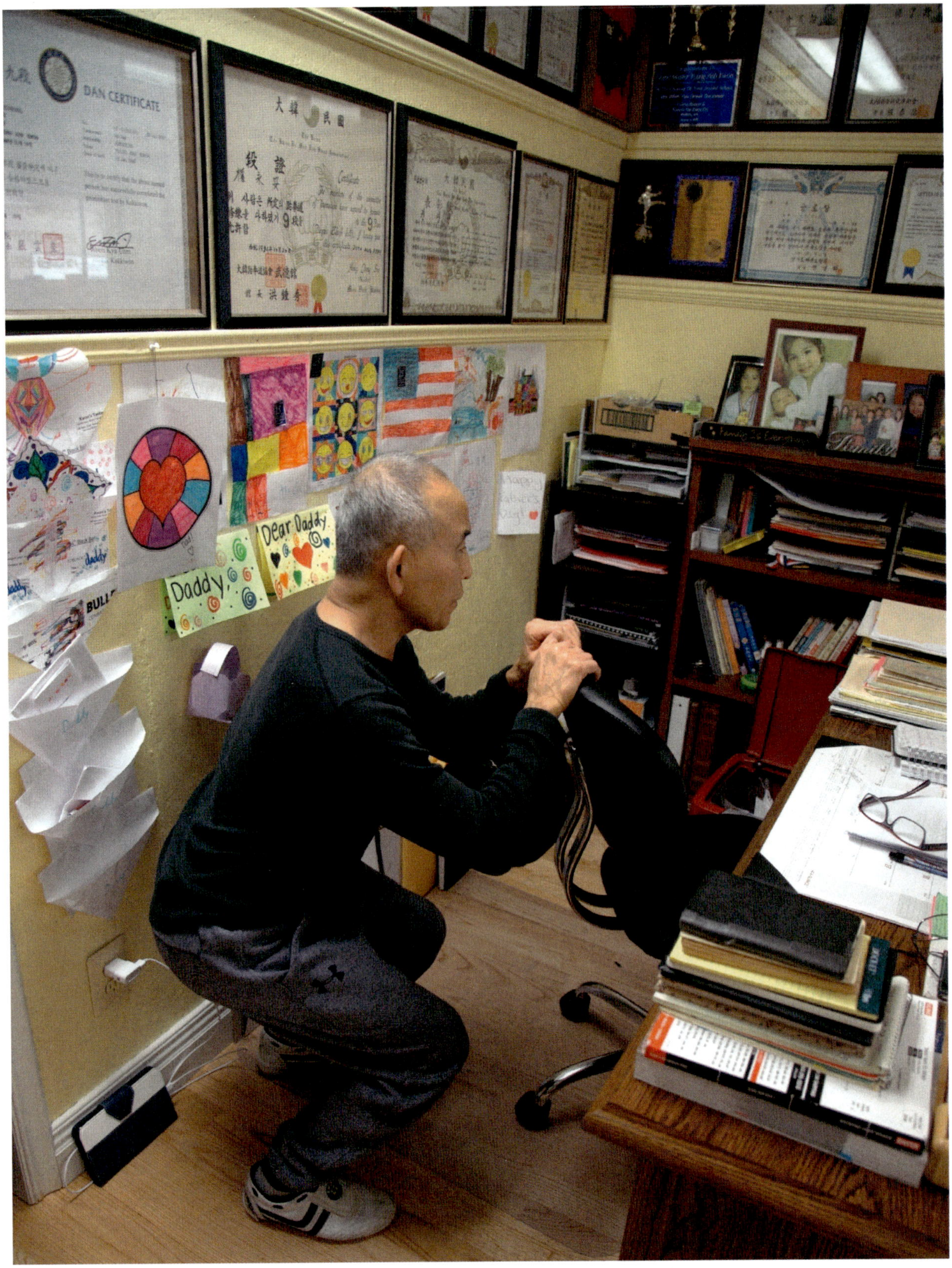
DAN CERTIFICATE
Dear Daddy
Daddy,

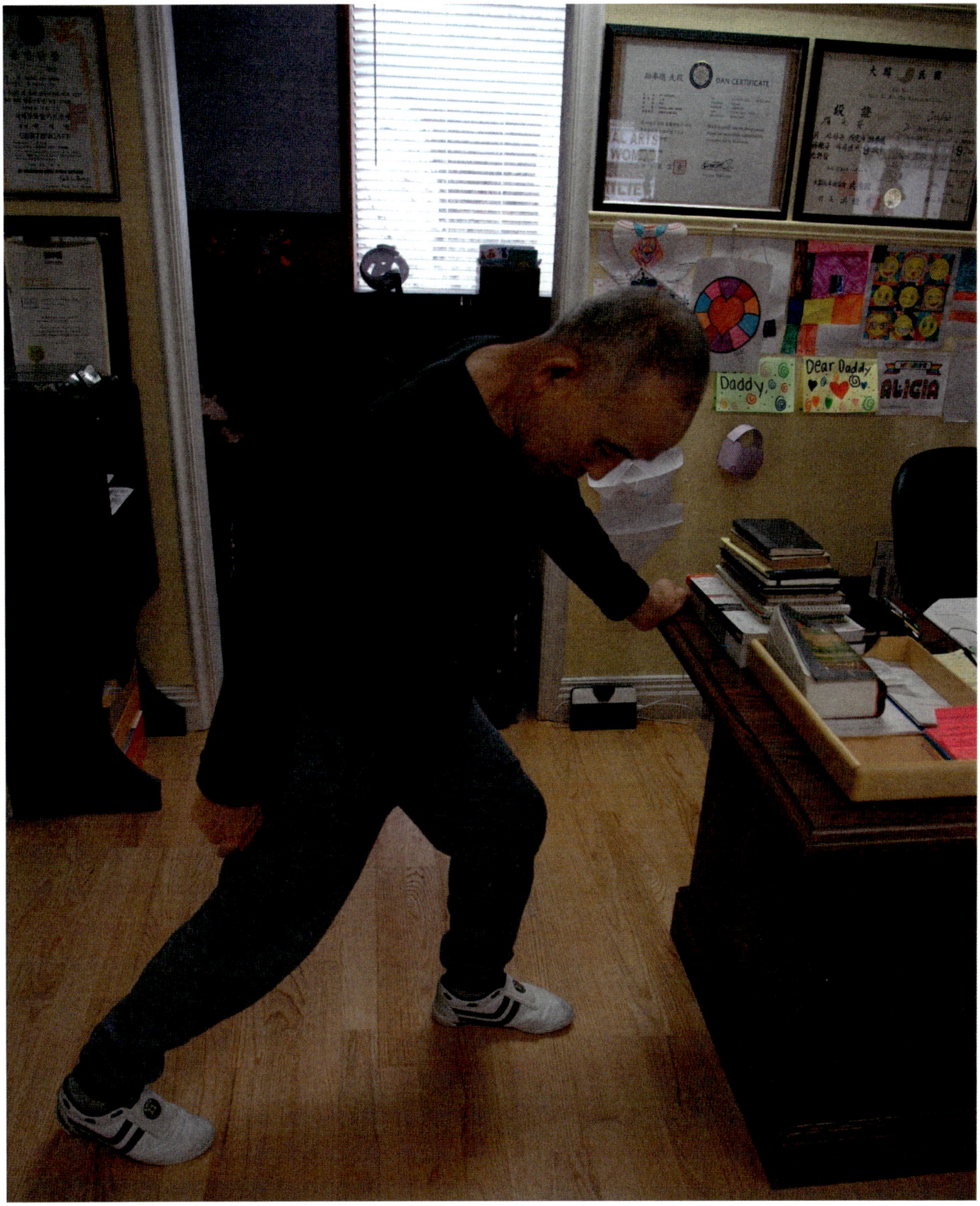
DAN CERTIFICATE
Daddy,
Dear Daddy
ALICIA

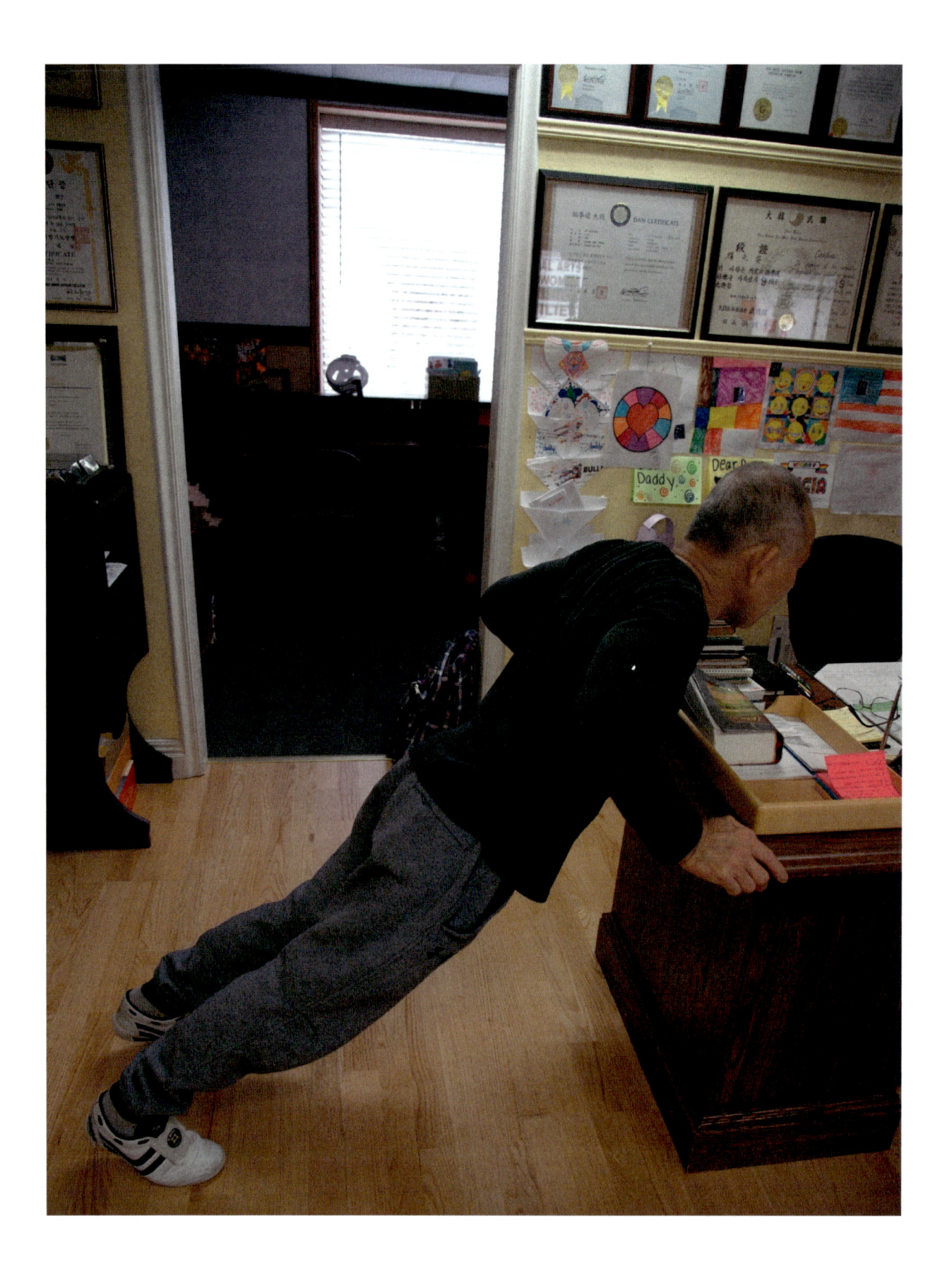

Walking

People only use a few parts of their bodies over and over. Most people only use 30% of their muscles. Using all your muscles will increase happiness. Some parts never wake up. The unused parts block energy flow.

To stay healthy, you must use every part of your body regularly. Otherwise those parts will get stiff and deteriorate. They will block energy. You want energy to flow easily through your entire body.

You can improve your health by something as simple as walking. We all walk in a certain preferred way, so from time to time, change up the gait. Walk faster or slower. Take small steps, then long strides. Walk backwards or sideways – anything different to put unused muscles to work. Swing your arms. As long as it is different, it will help keep you stay healthy.

If you use a stationary bike, sometimes pedal backwards.

Try passing a book from hand to hand around your body or balancing a cup while moving it around to put more of your arm muscles to use. Doing exercises to concentrate on one muscle isn't good if it neglects the other nearby muscles.

In Taekwondo, we kick a lot. Kicking the kick paddle at different angles uses all the muscles of the legs. In addition, it massages the feet. It is also important to work your fingers and toes.

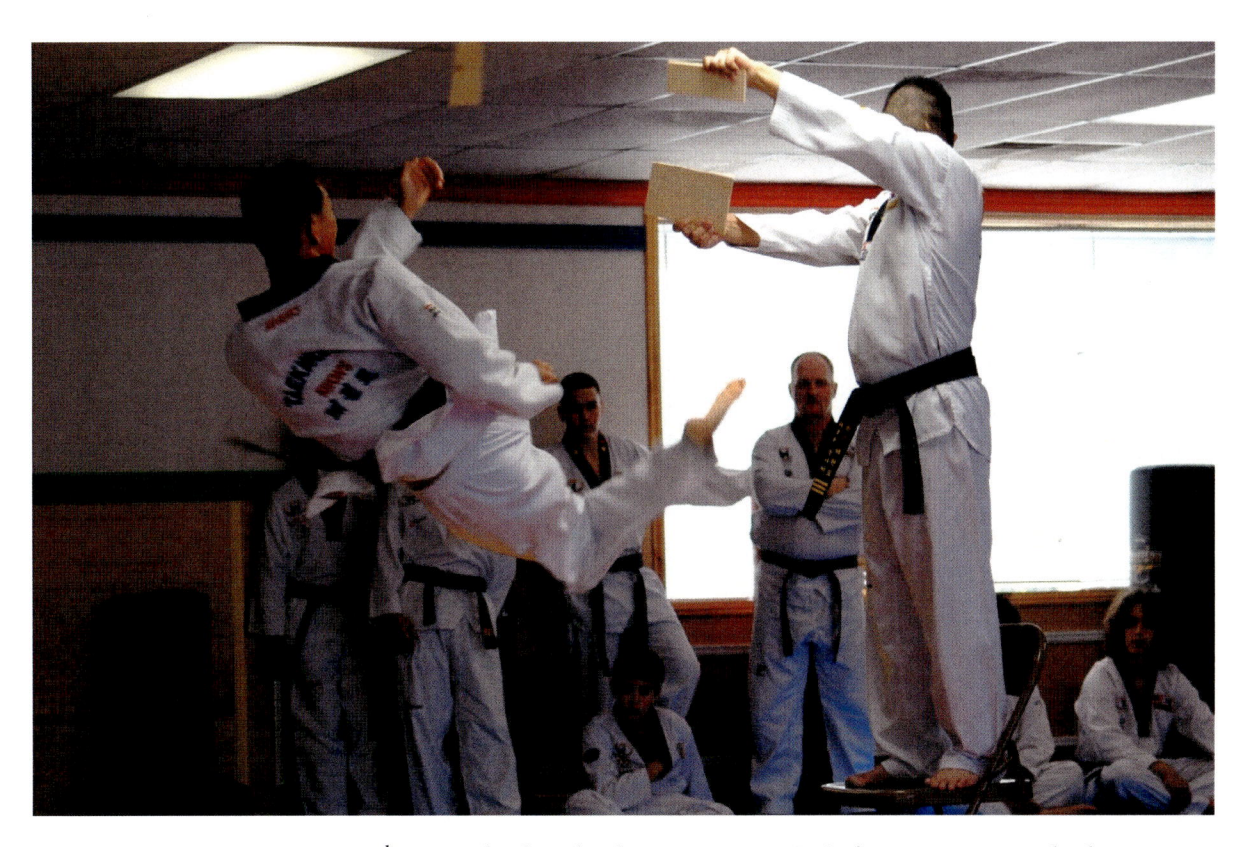

Son Greg Kwon, 6th Dan Black Belt, demonstrating 540 degree spinning kick

You also need physical contact to spread the energy, both good and bad. You can spread your energy out and into objects as well as people. This is one reason we do board breaking in Taekwondo, to train students to concentrate and to focus energy. It takes patience and perseverance to learn to focus energy effectively.

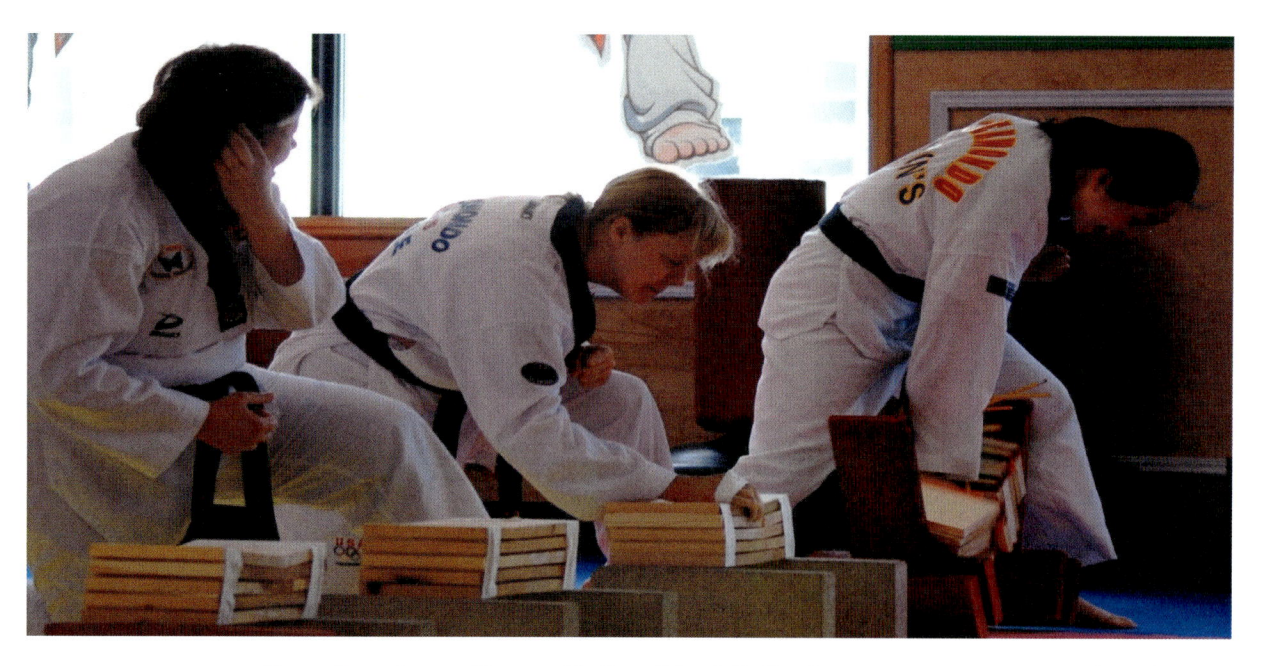

Daughter Jayne Kwon, 6th Dan Black Belt, demonstrating a power break

Trust and Confidence

The most important thing is to trust the technique. Whether it is the color diet, the exercises, or the massage, trust the technique! You have to allow time for things to work and have an open mind. Attitude is very important. Skepticism blocks the effects of even good techniques, but a healthy, positive attitude will get results from even a weak technique. It all starts with your mental attitude.

Breathing

Breathing can regulate the body, warming or cooling. We naturally blow on our hands to warm them on a cold day and blow over hot soup to cool it. Breathing is a natural regulator of the body. It is important to pay attention to breathing.

When you inhale, you take in energy. When you exhale, you release it. Control of breathing is important in controlling your energy, taking in good energy, and releasing bad energy.

The energy tank of the body is deep in the lower belly, just two finger-widths below the navel. You can calm your energy by rubbing your belly. Just putting your hands on your belly will stabilize your energy and make you feel better.

If you want to release bad energy, bad feelings, and toxins, you should exhale forcefully several times. It is very effective for lessening anxiety and anger.

To build up your own personal energy, you should breathe deep into the belly and hold it there for a few seconds. A very good technique is to lay on your back, inhale while covering your belly with your hands, and then squeezing your abdomen and pelvic floor while you hold your breath. You can do some shallow abdominal crunches at the same time to really stimulate your interior and get the internal energy flowing.

In Taekwondo, we use the *kihap* – the shout at the moment of impact for a strike or a kick – to focus energy. The martial artist stays as fluid as water and then – at the perfect instant – tightens his core and shouts as the muscles tighten to make the fighter hard as steel at the moment of impact. The *kihap* is very important and very powerful. It demonstrates the power of the breath when used well.

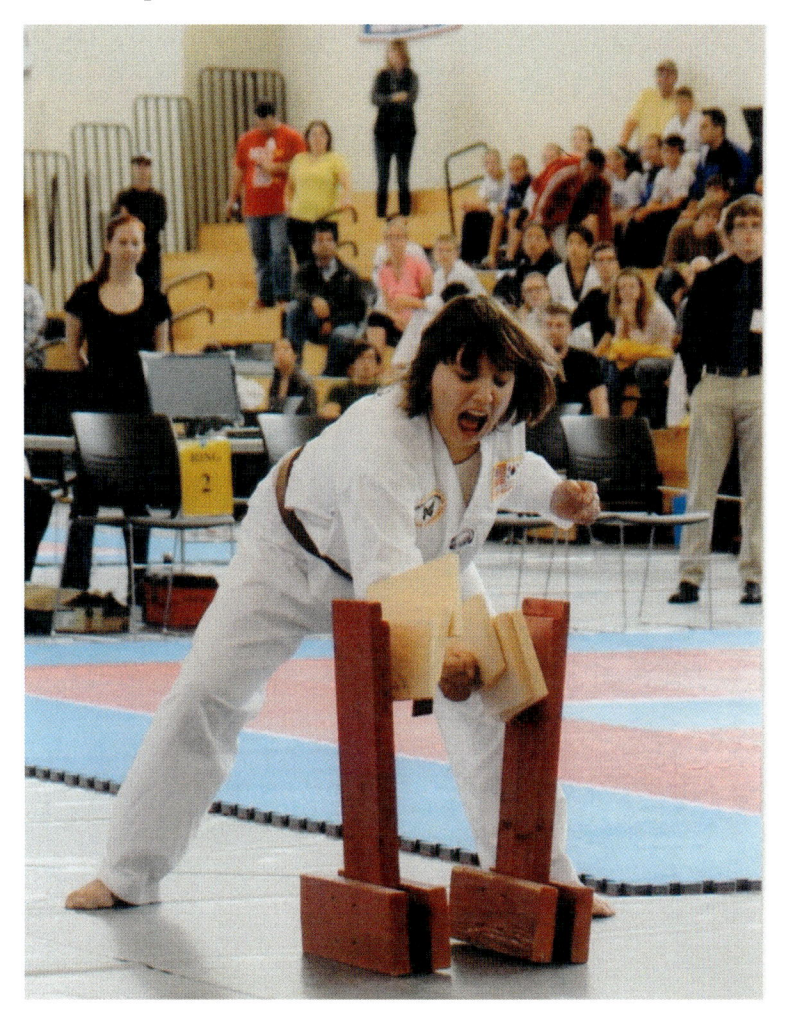

Kristina O'Donoghue demonstrating a power break with kihap

Older people dry up in the belly and become constipated. They strain at the toilet, holding breath, pushing their energy up to the head, raising their blood pressure. All it does is hold everything in. Instead, they should breathe to relax, lower the internal pressure, and let everything exit naturally. Straining at the stool is harmful and even dangerous. Many heart attacks happen from straining while on the toilet.

Holding the breath in this case is bad. It holds everything inside instead of releasing.

"As a kid growing up in the 1970s I saw martial arts explode into the US. I always wanted to train and see what it was like but never got around to it. So, in September of 2015 when I brought my son over to his Taekwondo lesson I was amazed to see people of all ages and conditions training together. The man leading the class was bright and motivated, full of energy and passion. I was especially impressed by his great way with handling the children, firm but kind and very encouraging, calling out recognition of the kids for a movement performed well (which the kids love). I was inspired that very day to sign up and take classes with my son. I met the instructor of the class who was none other than Grand Master Kwon himself.

I started training and immediately soaked it in like a sponge, however I had one problem. I was a badly out of shape 44-year-old. I had trouble keeping up with the class, easily getting winded.

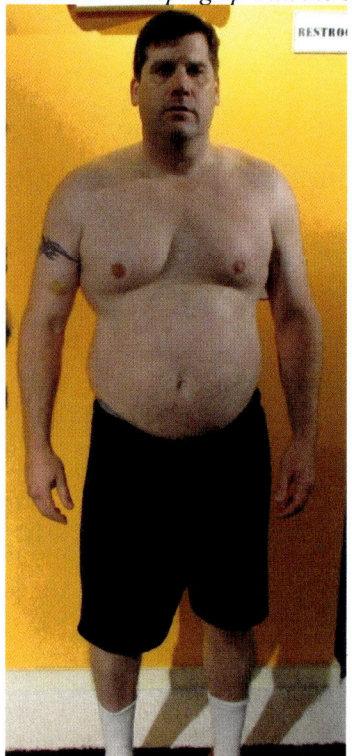

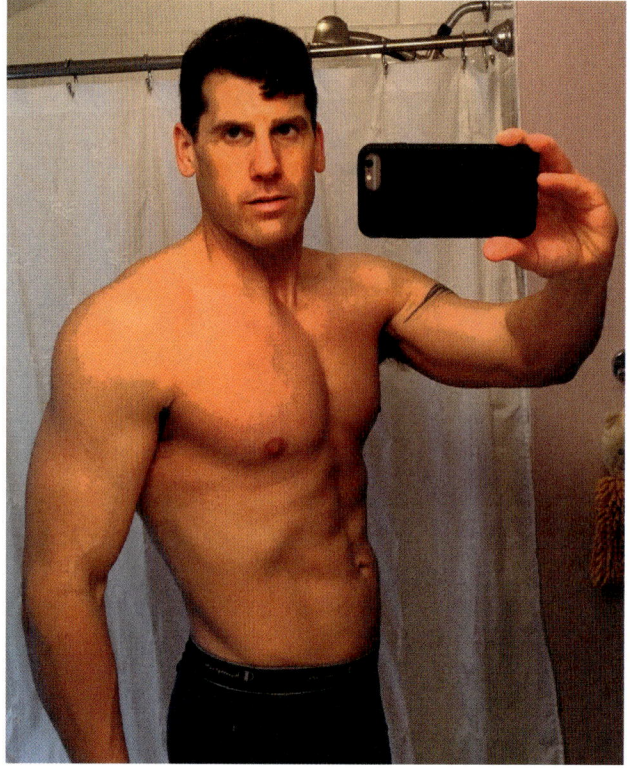

However, the environment and culture that GM Kwon has instilled at his studio is so positive and encouraging it never entered my mind to quit. His training methodology mixes cardiovascular conditioning with the Taekwondo techniques which forces you to get exercise while learning and keeping your heart rate up all at the same time.

GM Kwon has a way of finding some positive aspect of a student and nurturing that with encouraging remarks. For me it was board breaking. Although chubby, I was reasonably strong and could break lots of boards. He started calling me "superman." I became inspired to get myself back in shape so that I could do the same Taekwondo training that the more advanced students were doing, like spin kicks, rapid bag kicks, and other taxing training. I determined to do this starting in May 2016 at 265 lbs., 30% body-fat joining a local gym as well as continuing Taekwondo training. By July 2017 I have transformed into the best shape of my life at age 46, 200 lbs., 8% body fat.

There's something about training under the GM that lit a fire in me for fitness. I'm healthier and happier and truly feel lucky to have GM Kwon in my life."

~ Carl Soderstrom
Brown Belt

Energy

We are all surrounded by energy from the sun above, the air around us and the earth beneath us. Our bodies take in energy and store it. The newborn baby takes in energy through the fontanelle – the soft spot on the top of the baby's head – and through the feet. The fontanelle eventually closes, and the feet develop an arch through which they "suck" energy from the earth through the acupuncture point.

In the womb, the baby gets its energy through the umbilical cord and stores it in its belly. Even after birth, we still store energy in our belly tanks located just below the navel. You can increase your good energy by rubbing your belly, but it will also feed the baby if the pregnant mother does this, too. The energy tank – the *dan jun* – is the garden in which the baby grows.

Energy flows all around us and through us. When it is blocked, it doesn't flow freely, and bad energy builds up. It is very important to keep energy flowing, to bring good energy in through our heads, our breathing and our feet and to release bad energy. There are many ways to increase your own energy, for example by tight abdominal crunches, pushups or horseback stance while beating firmly on the tight belly. I learned some of these techniques from tradition, but much of my knowledge also came through self-experimentation.

Wear loose, comfortable clothes. Avoid thick clothing. Restrictive clothing, tight pants, neckties, or belts block circulation and hold bad energy in. Leave a finger's width between your neck and your necktie.

It is important to keep energy flowing through your body and to really feel it. You should massage yourself regularly by tapping and slapping your skin from the top of your head to the soles of your feet several times a day. There are several energy points on the surface of the body that can be used to take in or let out energy. For example, a sharp tap between the eyes will wake you up if you're feeling sleepy. There is a point on the sole of the foot that sucks up energy from the ground.

Before Bed

Sleep is very important. It is when your body rebuilds itself, so you should send the right message before you lie down.

Reverse the order of attention from waking up. Instead of starting with the feet and working upwards, start with your head. Tap your head and face all over.

Rub your face and around your eyes with firm pressure from your fingers. Hold your palms over your eyes and move them in every direction – up, down, and side to side. Say thank you to your eyes and notice how they feel.

Attitude of Gratitude

Gratitude is very important for health! Everyone should take some time every day to pause and say thank you to each organ and each system. Gratitude is a happy, healthy feeling and it will bring health where ever it is focused. Gratitude is essential to health and to happiness.

It is important that you check in with your body regularly. How is your body feeling? Are you hungry? What do you want? How do your eyes feel? How about your ears? Unless you check in with your body, how will you know when something is wrong?

Each organ is a life partner. Each body part works hard, but we don't appreciate them. Always be thankful for each partner. Saying thanks leads to happiness. Give them praise!

Be thankful to others as well. Have an Attitude of Gratitude and you will feel better. Helping others makes you feel good in the same way the other person feels good. If you give a drink of water to a thirsty person, you feel less thirsty.

Checking in with your body

After checking in with your eyes and thanking them, check in with your ears. Massage the ears, finishing with pushing a finger into each ear hole and pulling it out with a pop.

Rub around your mouth. Make a few faces – grin, grimace, and surprise. Stick your tongue out and move it around. Pause for a few seconds to say thank you to every part of your mouth – your lips, cheeks, teeth, gums, palate, and tongue.

This is a good time to "eat" some water. Keeping your neck straight with your head facing straight up like a baby bird ready to eat, pour a little water into your mouth and swallow it down. You will get air in your stomach, so burp it up. Burping is very healthy! It gets the noxious gases out of the stomach and makes you feel better.

You should roll your neck, shoulders, trunk and all your joints often and regularly. Joints, like metal machinery, will "rust" if not worked and lubricated regularly. And it's free!

Rub your neck and say thank you to your neck. Tap around your neck and shoulders, saying thank you to them.

Rub your hands and feet, between fingers and toes. Rub, squeeze and tap all up and down each arm, saying thank you to each muscle group and finally to your hands and fingers. Open and close your fists a few times.

Tap about your chest and upper back on each side as far back as you can. Then place your hands over your chest and say thank you to the muscles and then to the lungs deep inside. Put your hands over your heart and thank it for working 24/7 so you can live.

Tap and rub the *dan jun*, your energy tank just below the navel. Then rub around your sides and over the kidneys. Rub down the backs of your buttocks and thighs, then back up the insides of the legs.

Lie down and elevate the limbs. Shake them like a tree in the wind shakes out the dead leaves so new ones can sprout. When you have finished rubbing and thanking all of your body parts, you are ready to sleep.

If you think you are too tired to do this, you will not get a good night's rest and wake up tired. Good sleep is more and more important as we age. It is hard to develop new habits. It takes three months to get used to the new habits and changing circulation. Energy flow can be uncomfortable at first.

Chapter 4 – Food and Water

"Young Ahn Kwon is not only my teacher and my friend, but he is a second father to me. He is one of the most complex, yet humble and simple people I have ever met. We both believe that martial arts training promotes a healthy, balanced life style and gives the practitioner a respect for life and a desire to motivate others to live healthier as well."

~ Master Sal Fazio
6th Dan Black Belt

First, let me say that I don't like the word "diet." It sounds like a plan for cutting back on food or cutting out your favorite things to eat. I am going to talk about what to eat, not about what NOT to eat. Americans seem like they are always on a diet and always checking how much they weigh.

Needless to say, obesity is bad for health. You should keep yourself at a proper weight and not overeat. You should avoid smoking and alcohol. People should eat less meat and more fruits and vegetables.

I eat whatever I want and as much as I want. I weight maybe 135 to 140 pounds. I don't know for sure because I never check. What I do check is what my body is telling me. Am I hungry? What do I want to eat?

You should listen to your body and eat slowly so you know when you have had enough. If you eat too much, your belly will be unhappy. You can eat meat. You can have some sweets, even a little alcohol to celebrate a special occasion, as long as it makes your insides happy. Your stomach and intestines will tell you what they want and when you've had enough. You will know when to stop, but you have to listen!

When you eat, whatever it is, be thankful and happy. In many places, people do not get enough to eat and would be grateful even for some junk food. Eating slowly with gratitude will keep you healthy.

The Color Diet

I learned from my acupuncture teacher that certain foods have different energies. Some bring cooling to your inside. Some make you warmer. He recommended a diet twice a year that I always do. We can call it "the color diet." It takes nine weeks and is very easy to follow. It will keep you young and give you energy.

Purple

For three weeks, eat purple foods. Make sure about half of your plate at every meal contains foods with a purple color. Some examples are purple cabbage, eggplant, beets, purple-skinned potatoes, plums, and grapes. Some berries like blackberries as well as black cherries count as purple. It doesn't matter whether they are fresh, frozen, or canned, though fresh is always the best. Prefer the shiny, fresh vegetables and fruits. Eating half of your food as purple will clean out your body. You will notice and say to yourself, "Hmmm. Something is different."

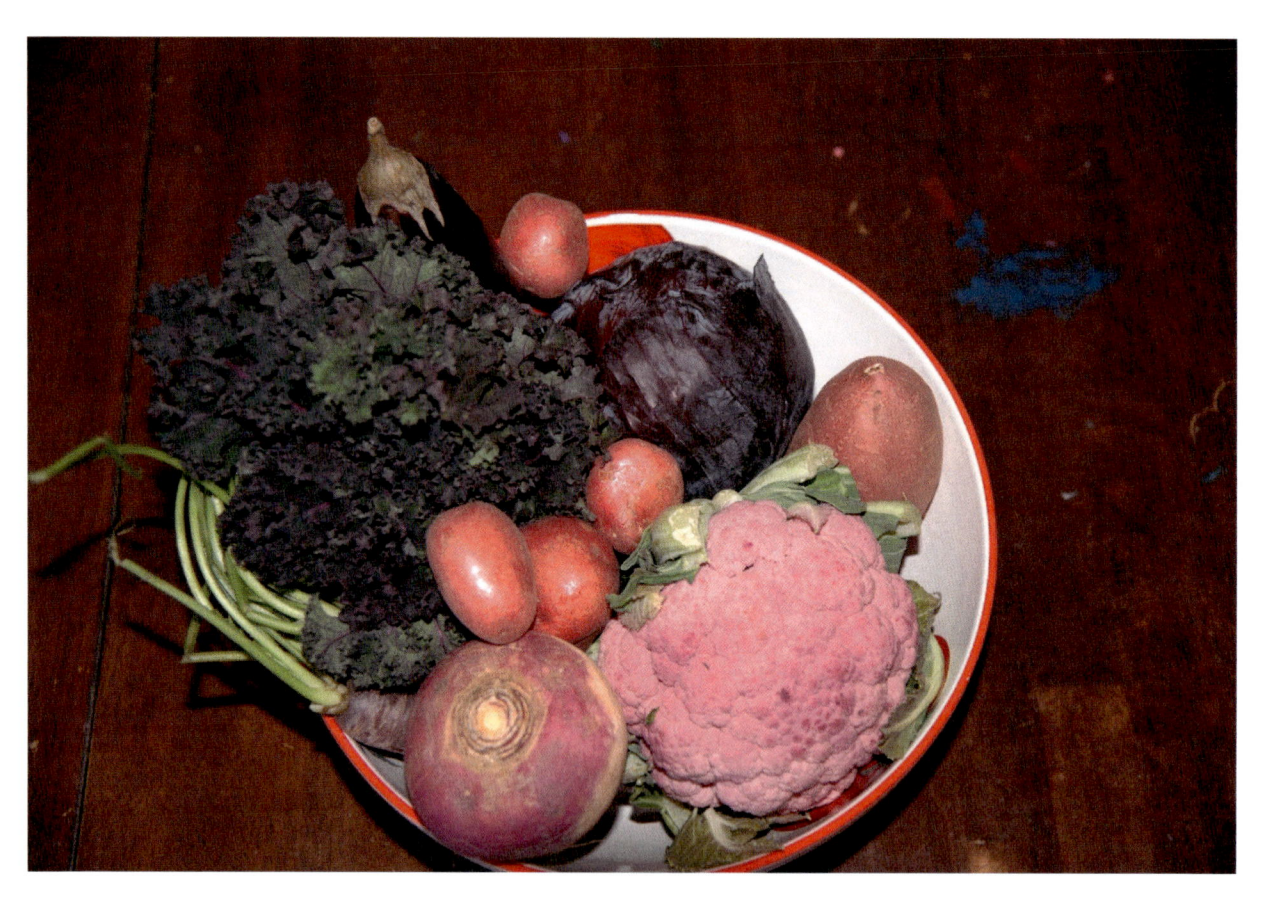

It is very important to pay attention to what your body feels like inside. Your appetite and energy will change. You may need to rest more often. You may need to cut back on some physical activity. Just listen and do what your body is telling you!

Yellow

For the next three weeks, half of your food should be yellow in color. Yellow foods include things like squash, corn, pumpkin, carrots, yams, apricots, peaches, mangoes, papaya, and oranges. Yellow foods break down the fat in your body and release toxins. Remember to listen to your body because you may feel different from before. The yellow phase is when people lose the most fat.

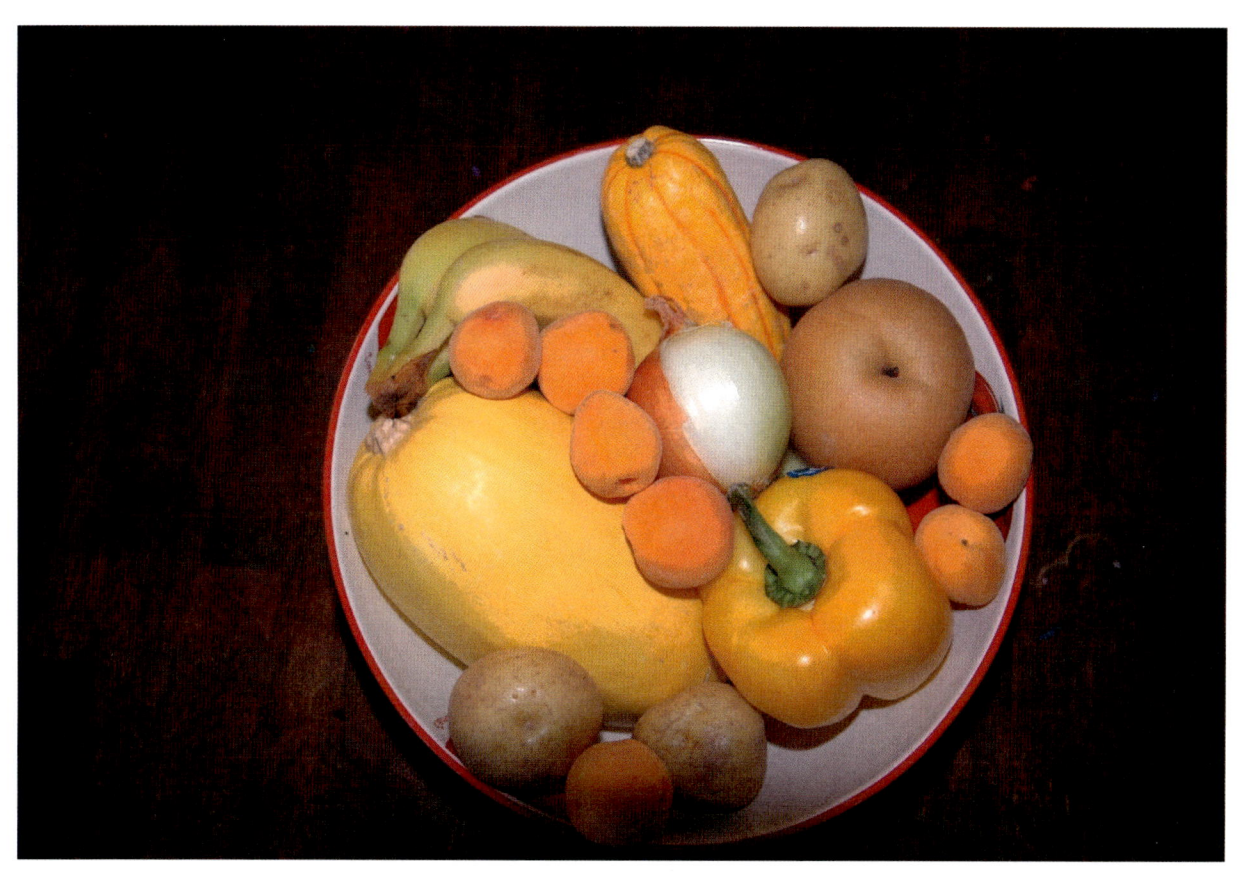

Sometimes people eat the yellow foods for more than three weeks if they want to lose more fat. That's okay. But be sure to listen to your body. When you release toxins from the fat, you may not feel well, but it will pass.

Red

For the final three weeks, you should choose red foods for half of what you eat. Red foods will restore your energy. You will be happier and eager to get out and do things. Red foods include strawberries, raspberries, cherries, tomatoes, red peppers, watermelon, and apples. You can also include some green with the red, like kale, spinach, and lettuce, and blue-colored foods as well like blue berries and plums.

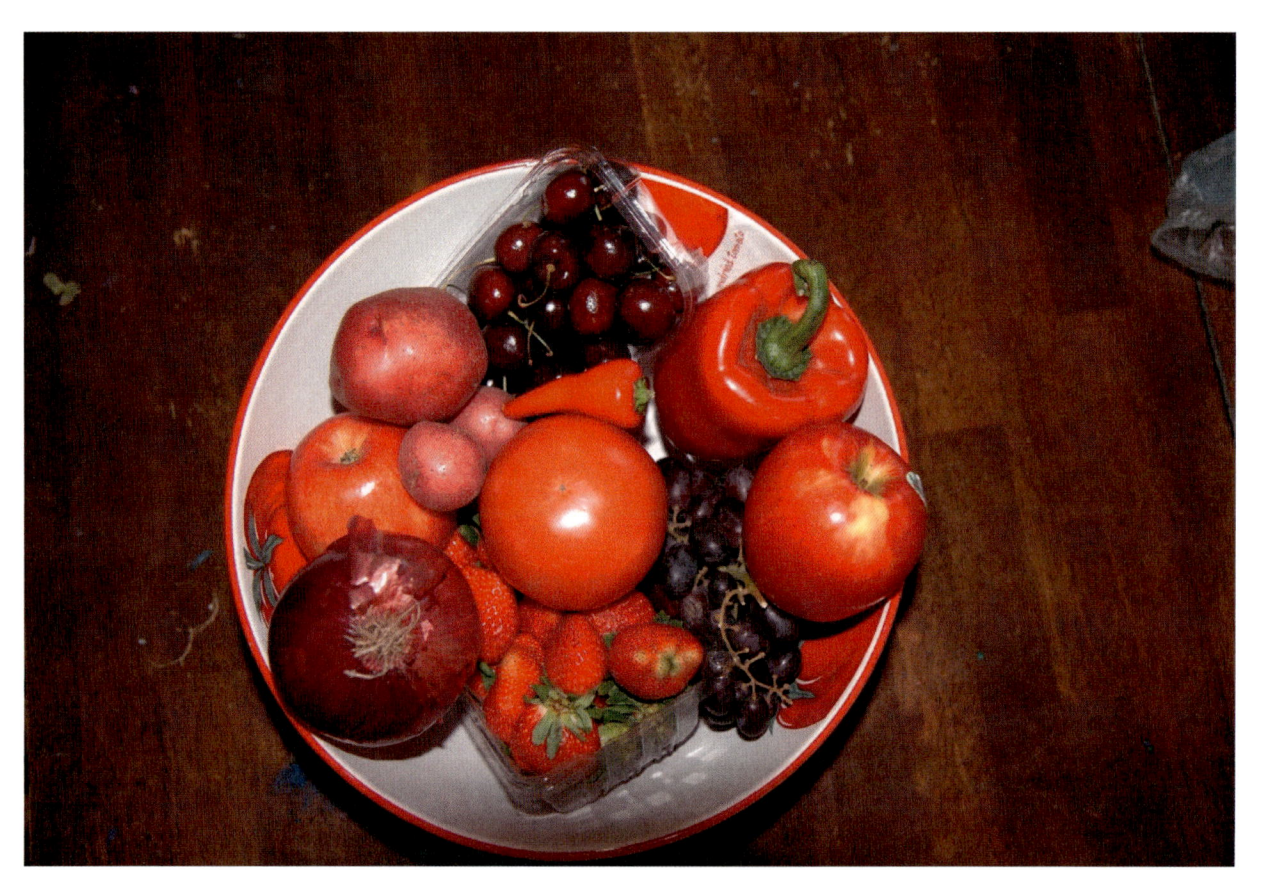

I also recommend that you choose a variety of foods. I try to get at least three of each color. This is not part of what I was taught, but I experimented on myself and it works. I think variety in food is a good idea in any case.

I believe in keeping traditions, but also in experimenting to find things that work better. Sometimes, you have to change with the times. All things change. You cannot count only on tradition. You must adapt. It is the same with the body. As time goes on, you must adapt to new situations.

I do the color diet twice a year, in winter and in summer. It is very convenient and always gives me good energy. You can do it more often and lengthen the phases if you like. For example, if you want to lose more fat, you could make the yellow phase longer. But you should do it at least once a year. Try it! It will make you happy and it will improve your health.

Water

Sip water throughout the day, not in big glasses. Big glasses of water all at once will make your belly unhappy.

From time to time you should "eat" water by pouring it into your mouth with your neck straight up like a little bird. Swallow air with the water, which will rinse the esophagus. The curves in the esophagus can collect bits of stagnating food, so you should straighten it out, rinse it down with water and air, and then burp the air back up. This will release noxious gas from the stomach and make you feel better. Foul gasses should not be kept inside. They will get into your inner organs and muscles, then come out through your skin and breath.

People ask me about water quality. As long as it is clean and refreshing, it doesn't matter. It is better to drink less than perfect water than to drink nothing, so don't be too choosy.

Chapter 5 – Lessons from a Long Life

"Kindness and compassion; our first impressions after speaking with Grandmaster Kwon for the first time on the phone. Grandmaster Kwon was immediately welcoming and offered our son Thomas a chance to start just shy of three years old! We decided to give it a try, not knowing how our family was about to change. Five years later, Tommy is about to test for his Black Belt, and our entire family of five attends classes every week. Taekwondo has become a cornerstone of our family life.

In the summer of 2014 our daughter Joyanna started the Tiny Tigers Program at 3 years old, and in early 2017 our daughter Marielle started also at 3 years, each after years of watching older siblings train. Grandmaster Kwon has always been amazing with the small kids, disciplining them when they need it, praising them when they deserve it, and letting them knock him over when they need a good laugh!

~ Liz Yennaco
Yellow Belt

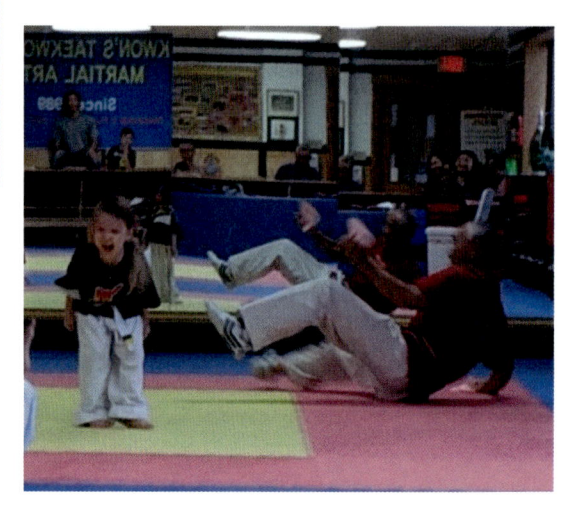

For a story to have a true happy ending, it must go through hardship. You must work hard to earn the result. You can't expect to collect anything of real value unless you work for it. Things that are easily earned are easily lost. Now, I am grateful whenever I encounter hardship. They are always an opportunity to learn and grow.

It is important to always be optimistic. Cultivate happiness, because happiness leads to health and a long life. Happiness and health come from inside. A good tree bears good fruit; a bad tree, bad fruit. It's the same with people.

Do not let problems get you down. Deal with problems quickly, then release them. Don't dwell on what you cannot change and accept problems as opportunities for personal growth.

Hobbies that increase happiness are important. They build good energy and lead to health. Many people like to listen to music, to play and sing and dance. I like golf and it is a sport I can share with my children.

Spending time with children will keep you young. Adults have forgotten how to ask questions, but children haven't.

"Grandmaster Kwon has helped our family in so many ways, including when our son was bullied at school last year. He instructed Tommy how to properly handle the situation and lead a positive discussion with the class by sharing strategies for how to deal with that difficult situation. Effectively, he turned a difficult situation into a learning experience for the entire class. That day our son left class feeling empowered, and we left feeling in control of the situation as parents."

~ Liz Yennaco
Yellow Belt

After Taekwondo training, check in with your body and listen. What is your body saying to you? Do you need rest? Stretching, perhaps. Or massage? Your body will tell you how much to rest and how much to train. You should make exercise a lifelong habit, so listen to what your body needs.

Always be training. Even at your desk at work, you can get up from time to time and do some stretches. Take a few seconds every hour to do a front stance on both sides and stretch out your legs, hip flexors, and calves.

The body is like a machine. It needs regular maintenance to stay healthy and live long. Good health leads to a good attitude and a good attitude leads to other good things. Bad health leads to sadness, which leads to other bad things. People should try to always keep a positive attitude and optimism.

The brain is the boss that controls the body – the CEO. If the boss doesn't take care of his employees, if he overworks them, they will get tired and give up. He shouldn't give them too much work and not thank them. You will eventually lose your balance of energy and health will decline.

We may not see it, but it is happening all the time.

People in their forties, especially males, suffer from declining health and sometimes die from stress. This is the age of most mid-level managers. They get pressure from the top and the bottom. They don't take care of themselves mentally and physically.

Stress leads to smoking, drinking, and eating junk food, which in turn lead to loss of mental and physical balance and health problems. When faced with stress, deal with it right away and put it behind you.

When you drive a car within the recommended limits, it performs most efficiently. If you drive too fast, you will wear it out, have breakdowns and accidents. People treat their cars better than themselves!

If you overwork your body, it will lead to stress, tension and anxiety. Energy gets blocked and balance is lost. You need to balance work with recovery. Small exercises with an open mind are very important. Balanced, regularly scheduled meals on a regular daily schedule are good, healthy habits.

Bad actions lead to bad habits. It takes a long time to clean up after bad habits. If you get in the habit of working straight through without getting up to move and stretch, your body will freeze in a chair posture. You will always be hunched over, bent at the waist, and look older than your years.

To make exercise a lifetime habit, you have to take charge of your life. Don't make excuses about how your job or your schedule won't allow you a few minutes here and there to train. It is hard for me to get used to how Americans talk. They always say, "Have a nice day!" You make your own nice day! You should say, "Make a nice day for yourself!"

Simply getting up out of your chair and doing a few stretches every hour is the first step toward being able to call yourself a man or woman of action. Don't just say a thing; show it! Do more than say "I love you." Show that you do!

(Next page) Poster for a Taekwondo demonstration to support families in need. Suwon, South Korea.

― 불우청소년 및 경로위선을 위한 ―
권영안 태권도묘기 시범대회

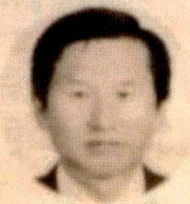

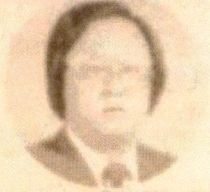

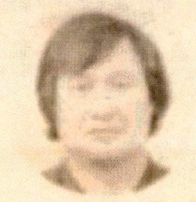

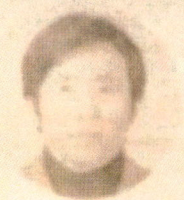

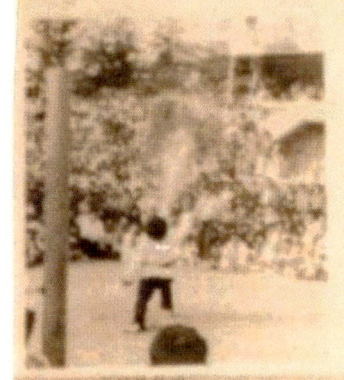

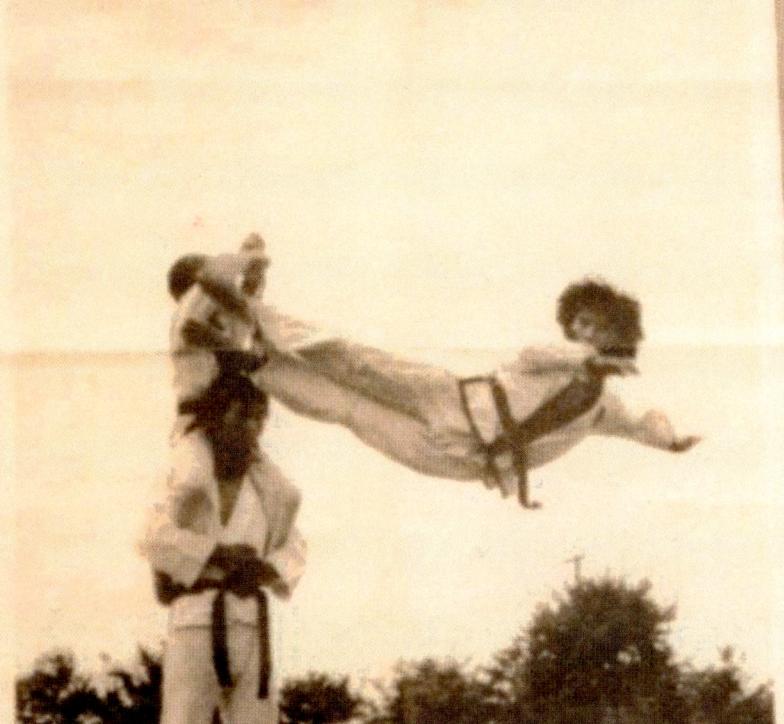

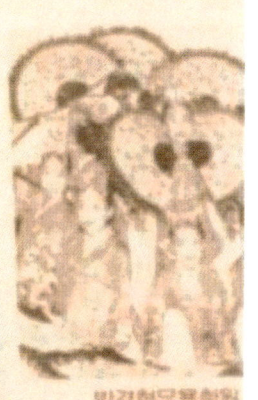

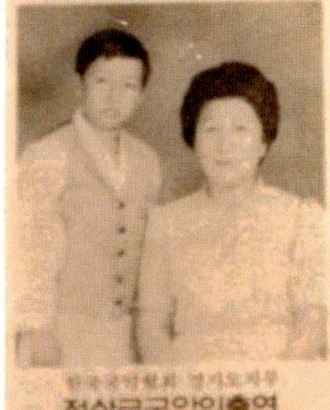

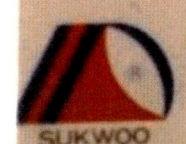

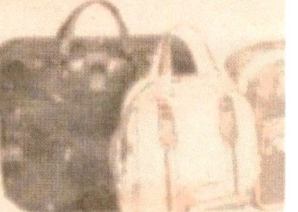

영예대회장 **최홍식** / 대회장 **이도형** / 추진위원장 **조근조** / 대회본부장 **권영안**

- 국가대표 어린이태권도시범단
- 과천체육관 건강체조출연

일시: 86.12.13 (토) 오후 3시 **장소: 수원실내체육관**

주최: 영안체육관 / 후원: 경인일보·경기도태권도협회 / 협찬: 창진운수주식회사

여행용가방·생활필수용품·거물생산품·단체주문 및 마출환영

석우체인가방종합백화점
☎ 6-2413

수원시 영동 5-7 (수원쇼핑옆 10m)

■ 예매처 ■ 경기도태권도협회 42-8074 / 파장동무덕헬스크럽 6-7100 /
우승체육사(남문역) 5-6189 / 무지개체육관(세류3동사무소옆) 33

Chapter 6 – Family Values

"We started classes at Kwon's Taekwondo when my twin girls were 4 years old – that was 13 years ago. They are now getting ready to graduate high school. Seven years after they began, my son, Anthony, was born. I used to bring him in his baby carrier while my daughters were taking class. He earned his black belt last year. We cannot say enough about how much we love Kwon's Taekwondo. As soon as we walked through the front door, Grandmaster Kwon has treated us like family – and that's what they are about – every Kwon's student becomes part of their family. They also learned about the Korean culture such as the language and proper etiquette such as bowing before you enter and before you leave. My kids are better people having been a student of Grandmaster Kwon. They now know it takes hard work and perseverance to achieve a goal, and also how to give and receive respect. They have become more confident now having the tools and skills Grandmaster Kwon has taught them."

~ Laurie Ganci
Mother of Black Belt

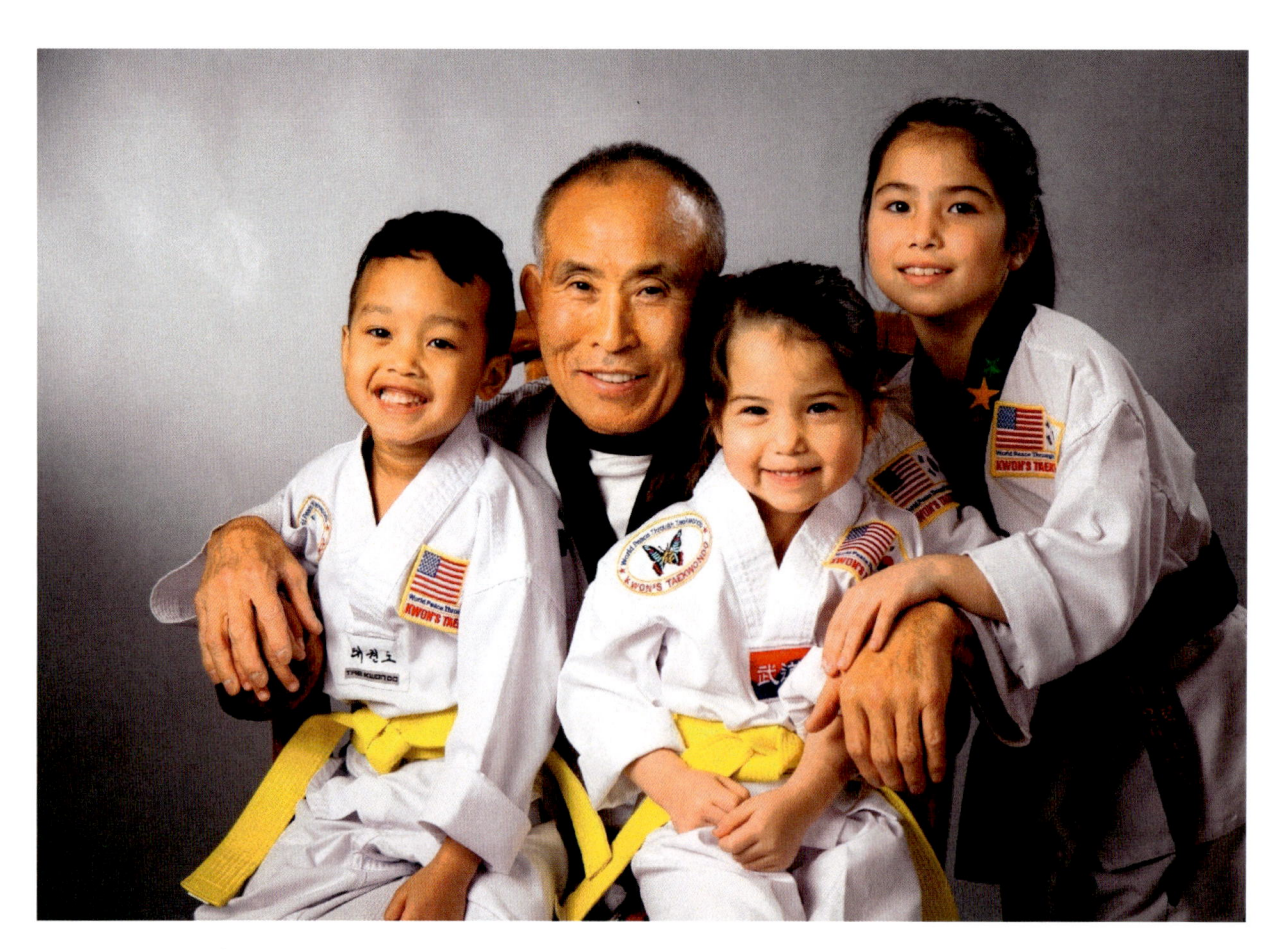

Grandmaster Kwon with grandson Kemson and daughters Alicia and Alexandra

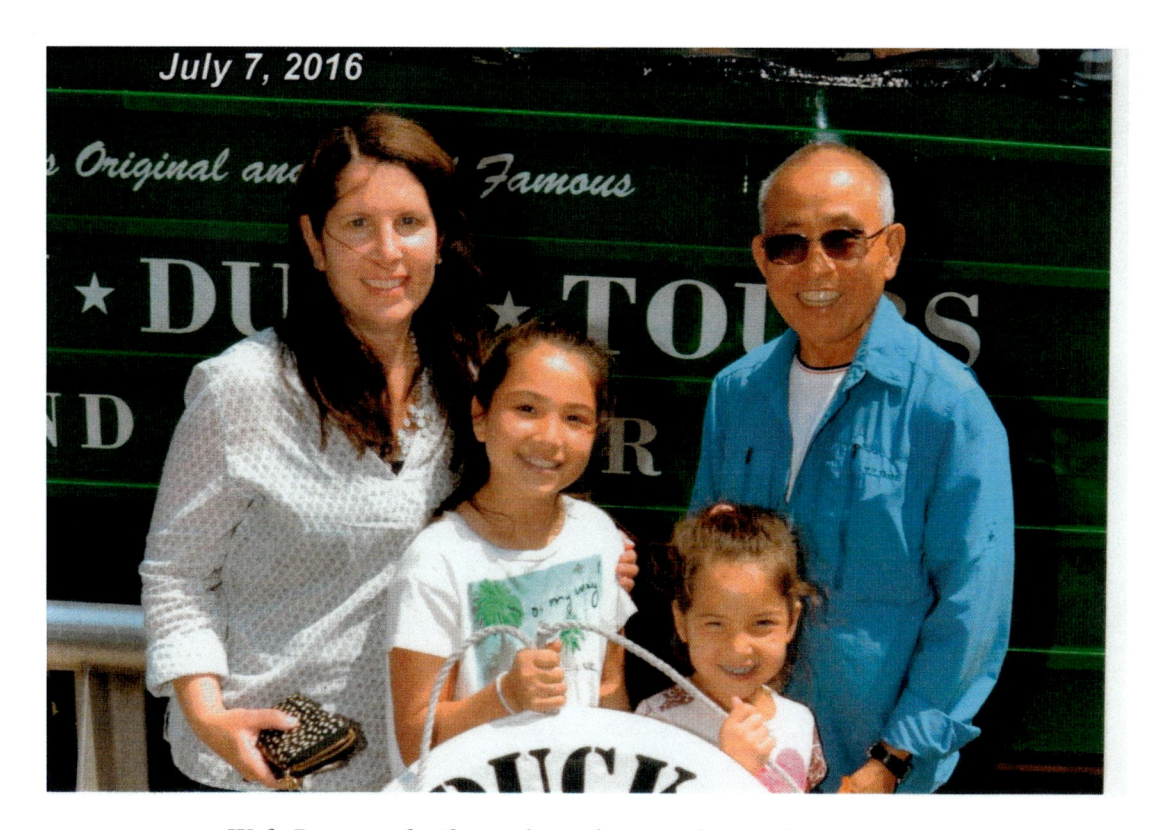

Wife Betsy with Alexandra, Alicia and Grandmaster Kwon

One thing that stands out about my school is that we focus on family values. I was taught traditional masculine values in Korea. Be a man. Look people in the eye when you talk. Be honest and trustworthy. Never hit a woman or a child. Show self-control and self-discipline.

Home makes the foundation for life. Just as good trees yield good apples, good families yield good people. In good families, good energy is freely circulating. Three fourths of education is at home, starting with the mother.

The mother is the first life teacher of the young child. In Korea, mothers carry their babies on their backs when they work. In America, mothers carry their babies in front, next to the heart. When the baby faces out, she sees the world. It is good for the baby to always be close to the mother.

By age six or seven, children begin to think for themselves. By the teens, they are exposed to potentially harmful things like bad company and drugs. A good foundation will help them make the right decisions as they become more independent.

When my school was smaller, I used to meet with parents of my Taekwondo students once or twice a year, just like school teachers meet with parents. At first it was hard, and I needed a translator. But it is very important for me to work together with the parents when training their children.

The main reason parents bring their kids to learn Taekwondo is for self-discipline and confidence. Second is for self-defense and exercise. You should not yell at or criticize young children. It hurts their self-confidence. I emphasize reaching out to children, using a soft voice and smile. I'm always trying out new techniques. I tell the parents, "For 50 minutes in the *dojang*, it's my kid. At home, it's your kid, but here, it's mine."

"(One) day he noticed our children were having trouble paying attention in class. As they were leaving he seriously called them into his office. They were relieved to know they weren't in trouble, but he told them they needed to work on their concentration. So, he gave them a "focus assignment" to count to 1000 and back down again on a grid sheet. This is another example of how he helps each of his students individually and treats us like family with the support we all need. Grandmaster Kwon is an amazing teacher, and we are honored and humbled to practice with him and to learn from him."

~ Liz Yennaco
Yellow Belt

Parents and teachers are children's guides to proper behavior. They must show, not just tell. They are role models who must set the example.

They should correct with a happy face, not with anger and a strong voice. They should never fail to encourage and praise for good behavior.

Children need firm discipline with a soft voice for balance. Mix challenge with encouragement. Sometimes I need to explain to parents what they are doing wrong. When it's their fault, I give strong talk to the parents.

Families are partners and should have a family meeting about twice a month. The family is not an obstacle to happiness. Be thankful and don't complain. Take time to think through problems and try to keep the home a peaceful place.

I give kids homework to develop discipline and then check their work. I even check myself! One exercise I used to do is to throw a handful of beans on the floor and pick up every single one. I did it to train myself in discipline, attention to detail, and perseverance.

It is not enough to do an exercise once and stop because you happened to get it right. You must practice your skills over and over every day until you can do them perfectly without thinking. I used to practice a different kick every month by doing 200 repetitions a day. One month it might be front kick. The next month, side kick. But the key was to perform the basic skill perfectly over and over again until any other way felt wrong.

Marriage

When difficulties in marriage come, be quick to change your mind from negative to positive. Always forgive and be the first to say you're sorry, even if it isn't your fault. If you don't, your health will suffer, and you must take care of yourself. Your health is the primary thing.

I gave my grownup children three pieces of advice about marriage. First, keep open communication. Always talk to each other and don't hold back.

Second, end disagreements quickly and don't hold a grudge. Grudges are rot and corrosion. They destroy the person who holds onto them and thinks about them over and over. Letting disagreements go and moving on is the healthiest thing you can do for yourself.

Third, never fight in front of the children. You should keep a unified front as parents. Support each other. Don't cut down the other partner to the children. This is very, very important. When the children are older and able to understand as adults, you can let them see your disagreements, but not when they are young. They won't understand, and it will upset them. Children need a stable, safe home where they can feel that both parents love them and are committed to their well-being. When dealing with others, including your partner, show self-control and self-discipline. Children learn by example.

When you make a promise to a child, always keep it. It is more important to them than it is to you. If you don't keep your promises, they will learn that keeping promises isn't important.

Don't show anger to children. Children see you as an example. What you give comes back to you multiplied many times. So, always be nice to your partner, your children and other people and send out good energy. You will always sleep well if you do.

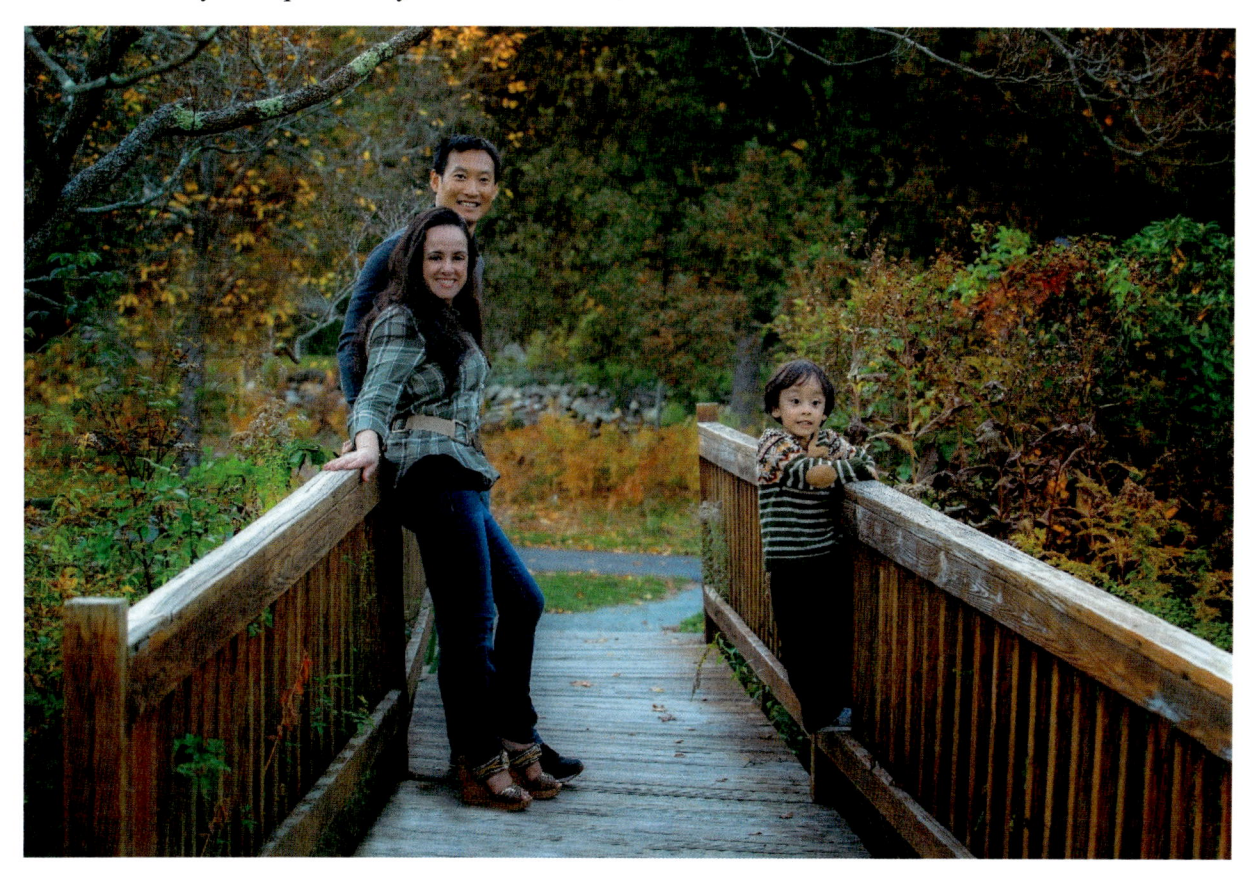

Master Greg Kwon, his wife Diva and son Angelo

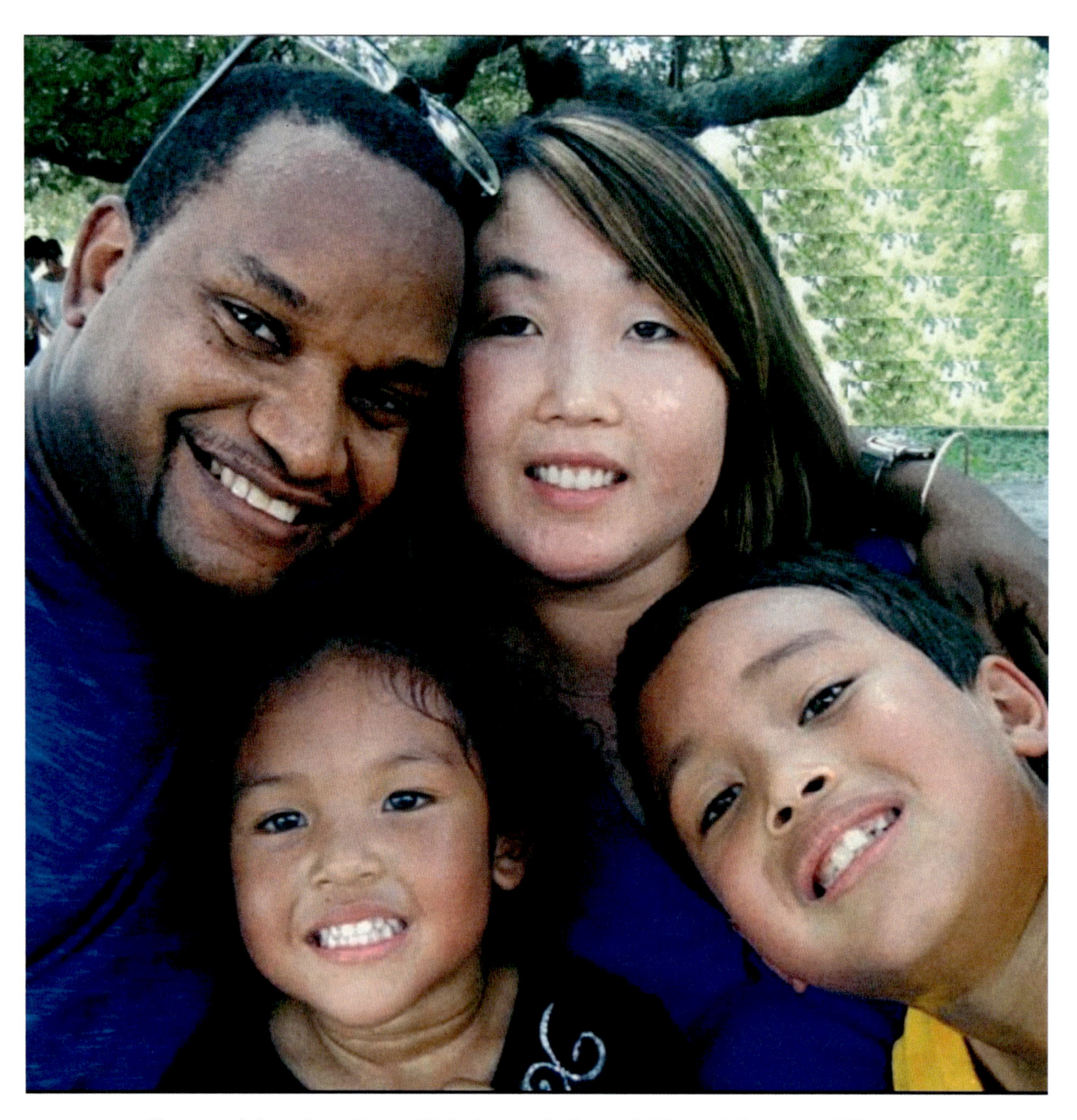

Ikem and daughter Jayne Ugbolue with their children Adaora and Kemson

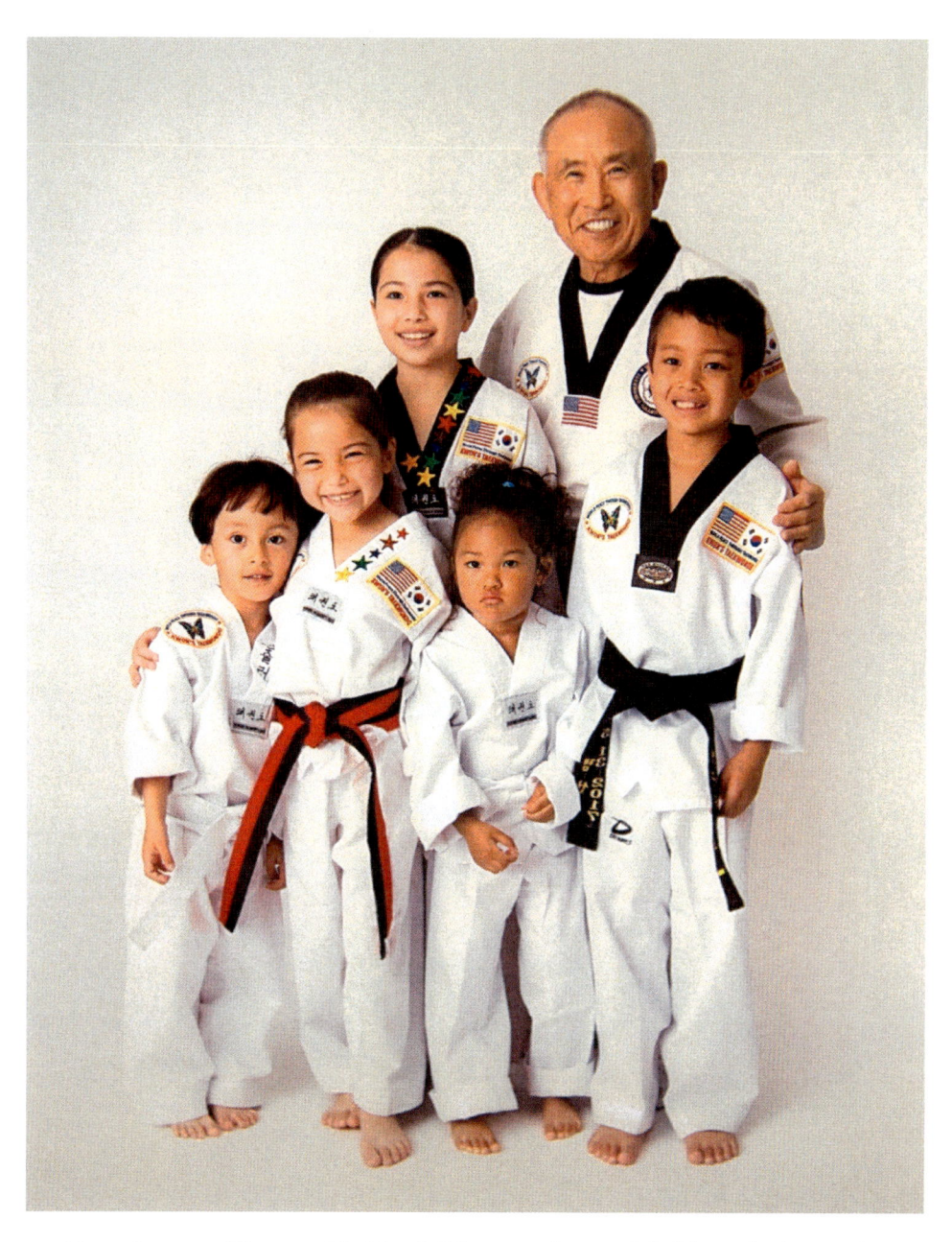

Grandmaster Kwon with his children and grandchildren, left to right:

Angelo, Alicia, Alexandra, Adaora and Kemson

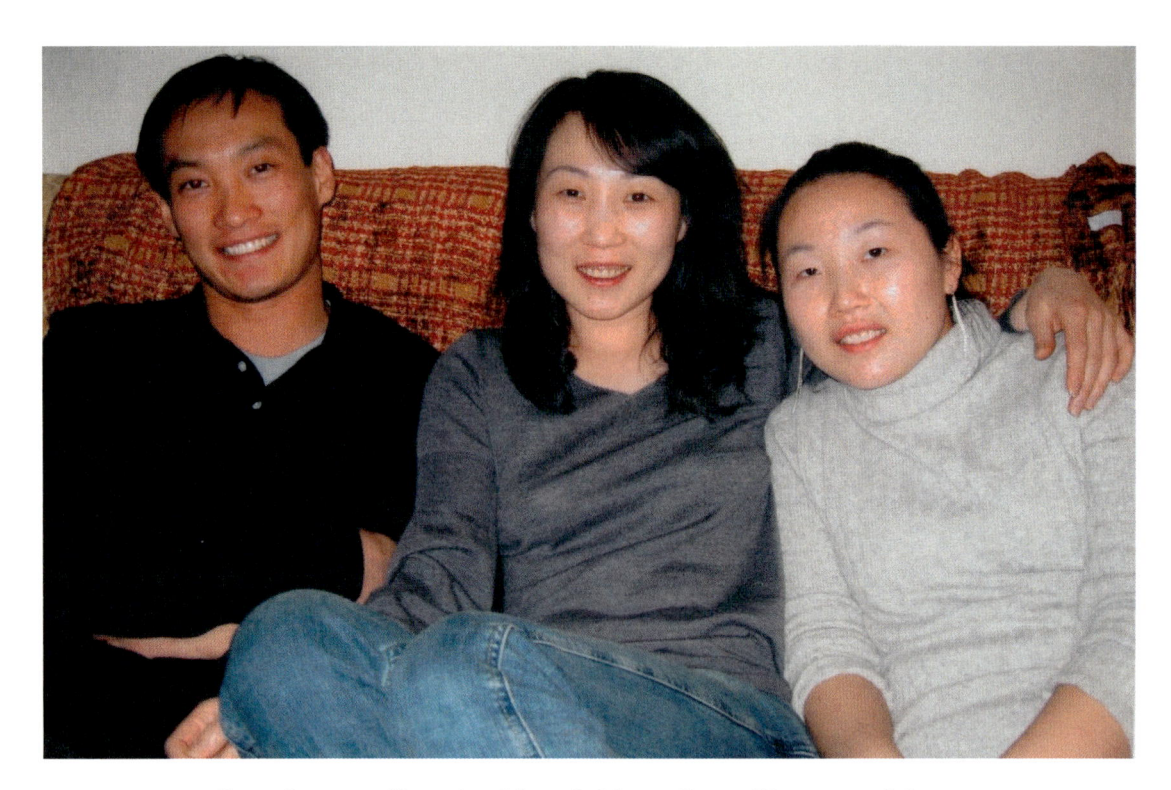

Grandmaster Kwon's older children Greg, Hoejin and Jayne

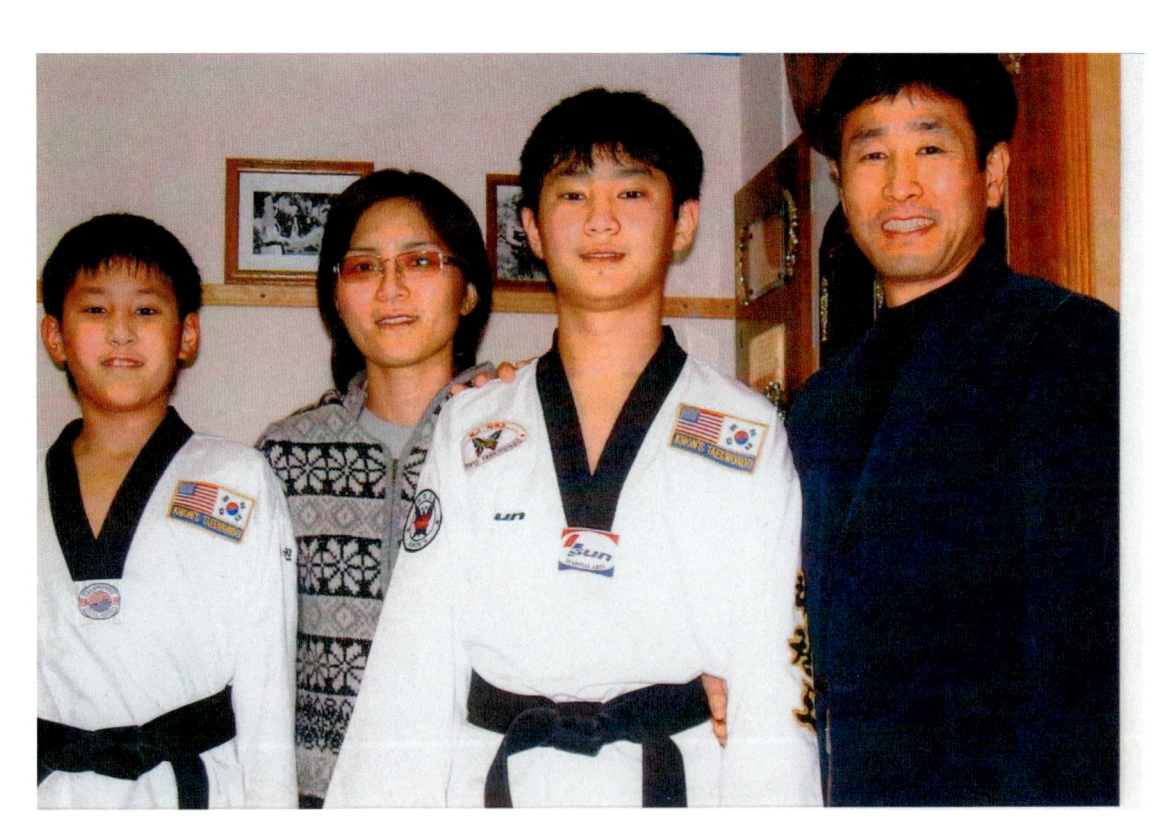

Grandmaster Kwon's brother Richard (right) with his family

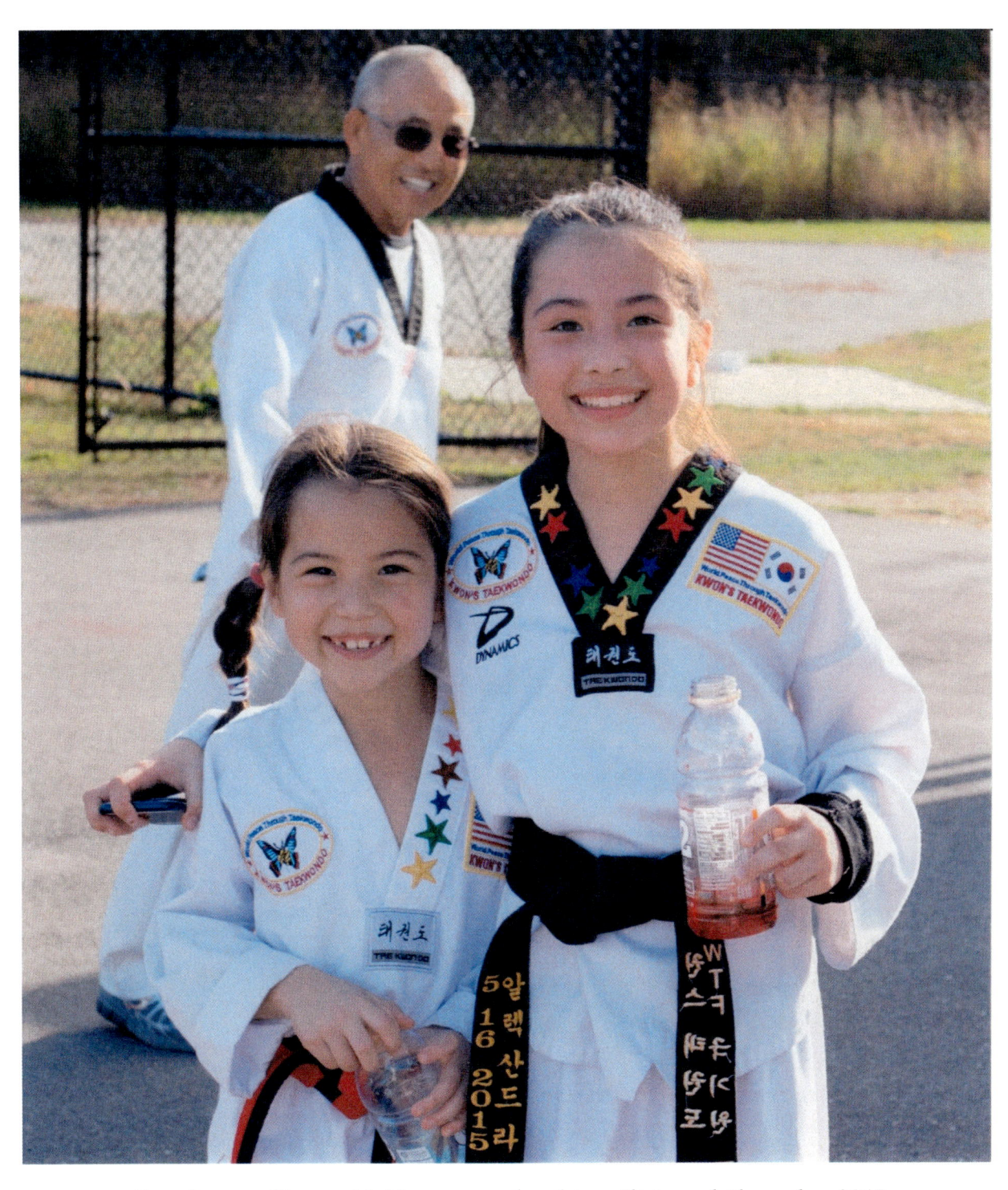

Grandmaster Kwon with his younger daughters Alicia and Alexandra, 2017

Chapter 7 – Taekwondo

"I came to Grand Master Kwon's school following the completion of my son's chemotherapy treatment. I could see that after two years of treatment that it had a definite impact on his overall physicality. I believe, this in turn affected his confidence and daringness to challenge himself. Because TKD offers a more self-paced approach, I thought it would be an excellent way to build my son, Liam, back up.

After looking at several schools, I came into Kwon's TKD, Grand Master Kwon's dojang. I could tell in five minutes of being there that it was the right place for my son. Grand Master Kwon was involved in every class and struck the proper balance between discipline and fun. In my experience, it is rare to see a 9th Dan this involved in all the classes and I felt lucky to come upon his school.

After several months of training, I could see improved coordination and increased strength. I could see Liam start to regain confidence in himself and wanting to challenge himself more.

My son loved to break boards and was always looking for an opportunity to practice his technique. Liam performed breaking in his regular school as part of a talent day event. This was a huge deal for Liam as he was now center stage in front of his fellow students. Liam performed his techniques without a hiccup and broke all his boards. He was beaming with pride and accomplishment.

Liam has gone on to play many other sports such as baseball, basketball, and even football. He approaches each experience with a winning spirit and drive to improve himself to his own capabilities. I believe these are the foundational building blocks that are the core to Grand Master Kwon's school.

It wasn't long after my son started taking classes that I decided to pick up where I left off in my own TKD training. I've been training at Grand Master Kwon's dojang for over five years."

~ Kevin Flynn
3rd Dan Black Belt

"Grandmaster Young Ahn Kwon is someone who has had an immeasurable impact on the taekwondo community. Known for his integrity, his emphasis on family values, and of course his outstanding martial arts, Grandmaster Kwon is someone who shines as a giant in his field and who has the respect of everyone who knows him. He has spent a lifetime thinking about the mechanics and health of the human body."

~ Master Dan Chuang
Head Instructor, CW Taekwondo at Boston
Head Instructor, MIT Sport Taekwondo Club
Head Coach, USA National Poomsae Taekwondo Team

All beings – even animals – are born with natural defenses. Think of skunks, bees, and porcupines. When attacked, we all have a natural instinct to move away from the threat and protect ourselves.

Taekwondo began when people began, at the dawn of the human race. It started with natural movements which are a part of everyday life. Taekwondo techniques – blocks, strikes and kicks – originated from movements that were basic for protection and meeting basic needs. They developed from everyday experiences. Natural movements were improved upon to become specific techniques that were better.

All martial arts require practice, practice, practice! It takes years for a student to learn all of the basic techniques of Taekwondo and earn a first-degree black belt, or 1st Dan. There is also a junior black belt, or *poom*, for kids below the age of 16, so it is never too early to start.

The black belt test is very challenging for any age and takes four days. The student must demonstrate all of the basic kicks, strikes and blocks, skill at sparring, basic self-defense, and all eight of the basic *poom sae*. On one of the test days, the students must run three miles and do 500 pushups and 500 sit-ups to demonstrate physical fitness.

After earning a black belt, more highly advanced *poom sae* must be mastered and the self-defense techniques are more demanding. Of course, you cannot just forget the eight basic *poom sae* and leave them behind, either. After practicing as a black belt for at least three years and perfecting your techniques, you may rise to the level of 3rd dan, or Instructor. At this level, you can teach independently at an accredited school.

Seven years after earning 3rd dan, a Taekwondo instructor may reach the level of Master, or 5th dan. By this level, a person is already dedicated to Taekwondo for life.

Beyond 5th dan lie 8th and 9th dan, the levels of the grandmaster. If you think of a black belt as a high school diploma and 3rd dan as a bachelor's degree, then 5th dan is a master's degree and the grandmaster level is a PhD, except that there are much fewer grandmasters than PhDs in the world. At this writing, only 86 people have ever reached the level of 9th dan in the United States. About 15 to 20 percent of them are no longer alive.

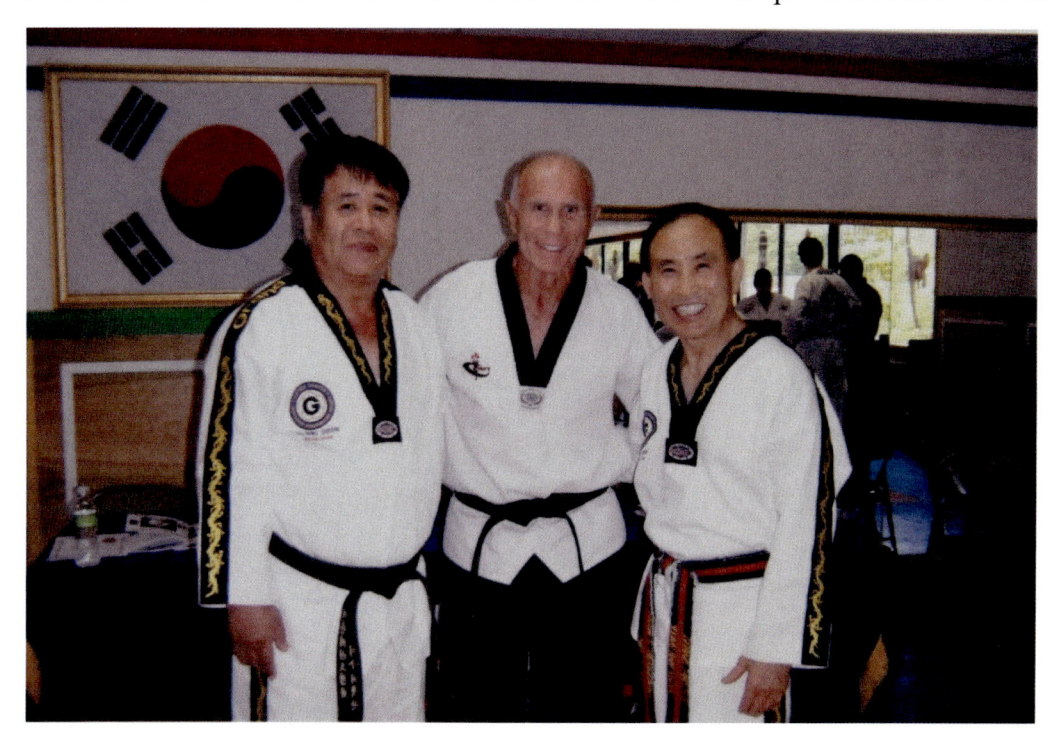

Grandmaster Tae Byung Park, Bill "Superfoot" Wallace, Grandmaster Kwon

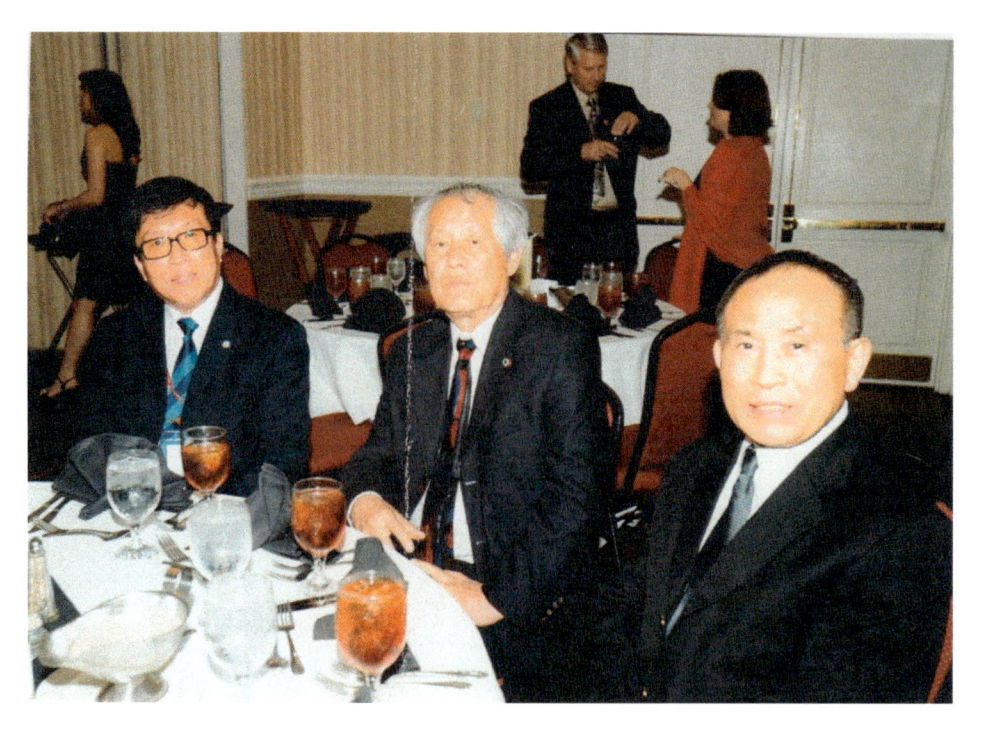

Grandmasters Heang Ki Paik, Woo Jin Jung and Young Ahn Kwon

There are 210 countries with 80 million people that practice Taekwondo today. Because Taekwondo is an international sport, it can also be a vehicle for diplomacy. In 2011 we hosted the North Korean National Taekwondo Demonstration Team. It was the second time the Taekwondo community in America was able to make this amazing event happen.

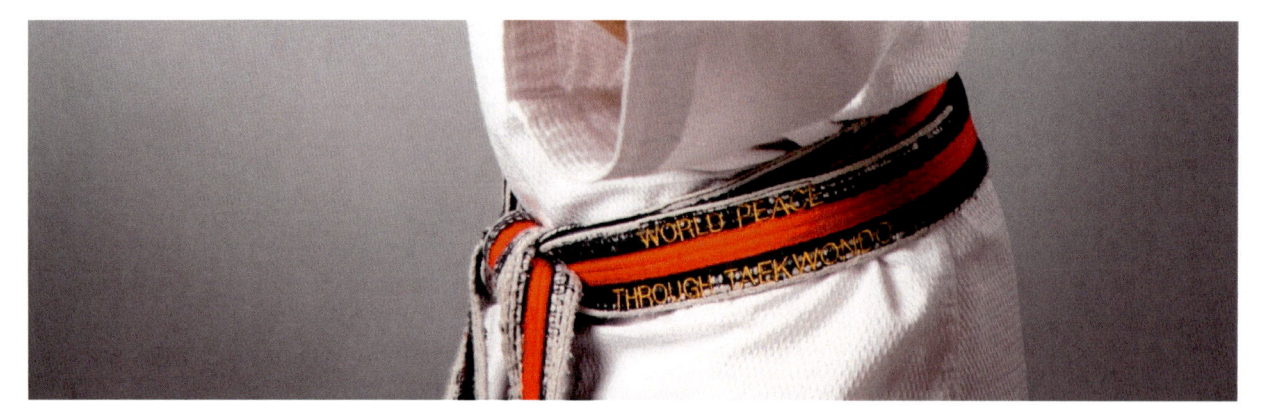

The words "World Peace Through Taekwondo" are on my belt and I believe in it with all my heart!

Goodwill Tour 2011

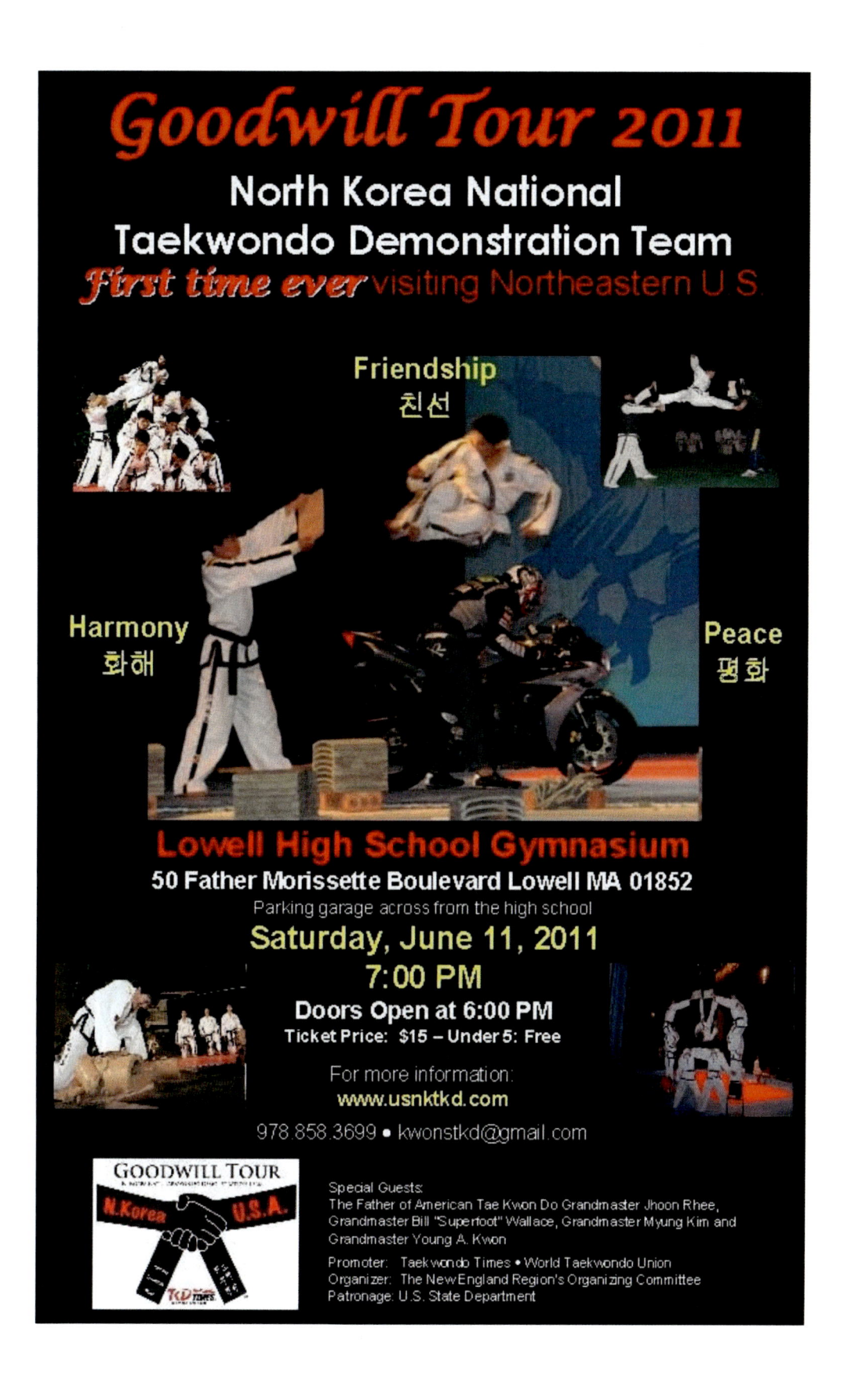

North Korea National Taekwondo Demonstration Team

First time ever visiting Northeastern U.S.

Friendship 친선

Harmony 화해

Peace 평화

Lowell High School Gymnasium
50 Father Morissette Boulevard Lowell MA 01852

Parking garage across from the high school

Saturday, June 11, 2011
7:00 PM
Doors Open at 6:00 PM
Ticket Price: $15 – Under 5: Free

For more information:
www.usnktkd.com

978.858.3699 • kwonstkd@gmail.com

Special Guests:
The Father of American Tae Kwon Do Grandmaster Jhoon Rhee, Grandmaster Bill "Superfoot" Wallace, Grandmaster Myung Kim and Grandmaster Young A. Kwon

Promoter: Taekwondo Times • World Taekwondo Union
Organizer: The New England Region's Organizing Committee
Patronage: U.S. State Department

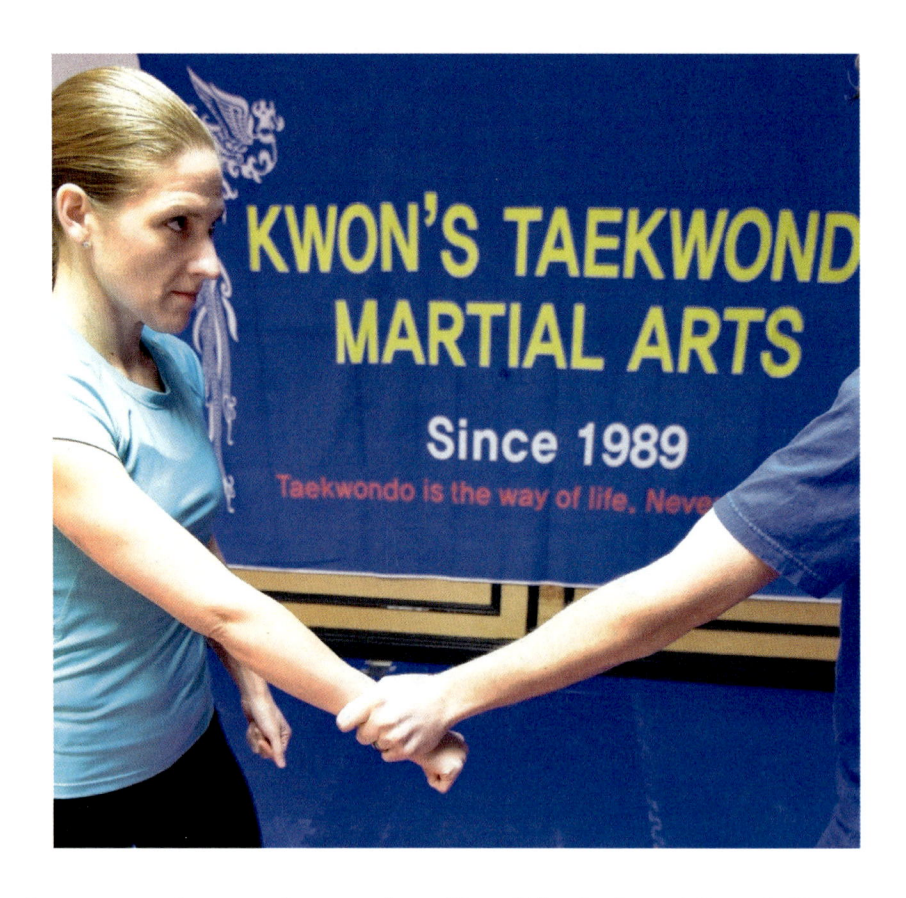

In our self-defense classes, couples practice together. Here Elizabeth and Joseph Yennaco rehearse a response to an unwanted wrist grab.

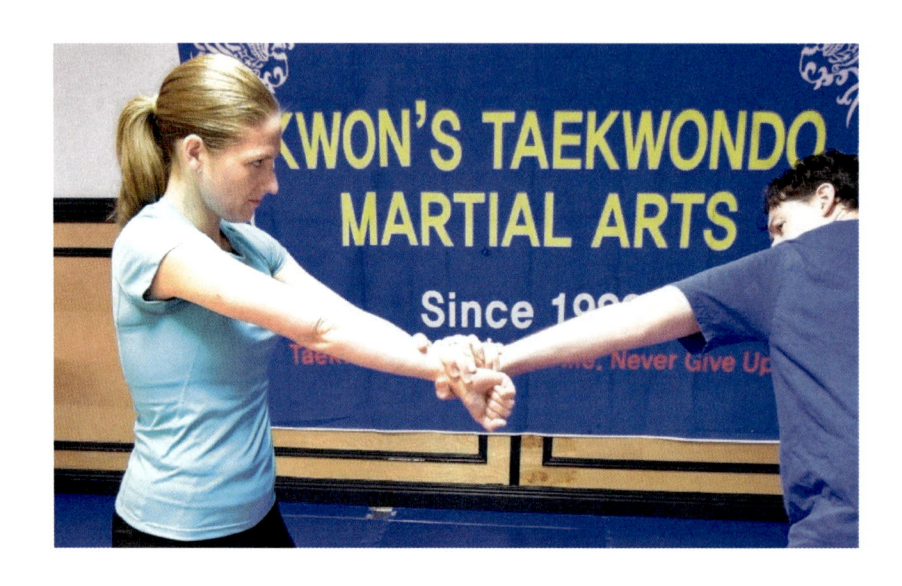

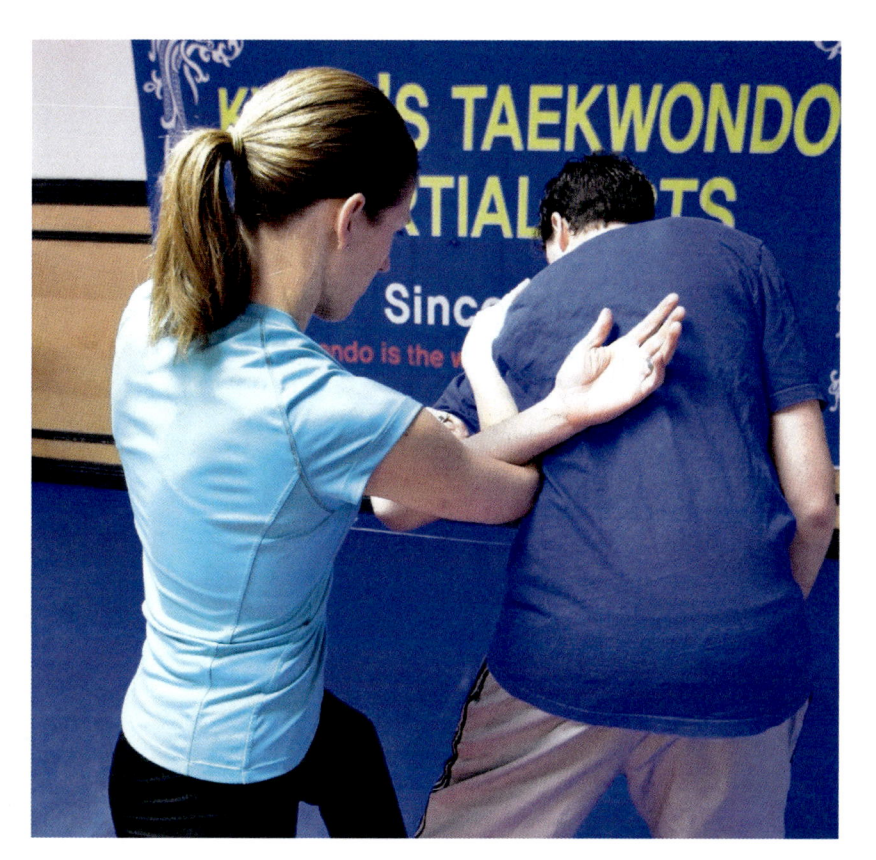

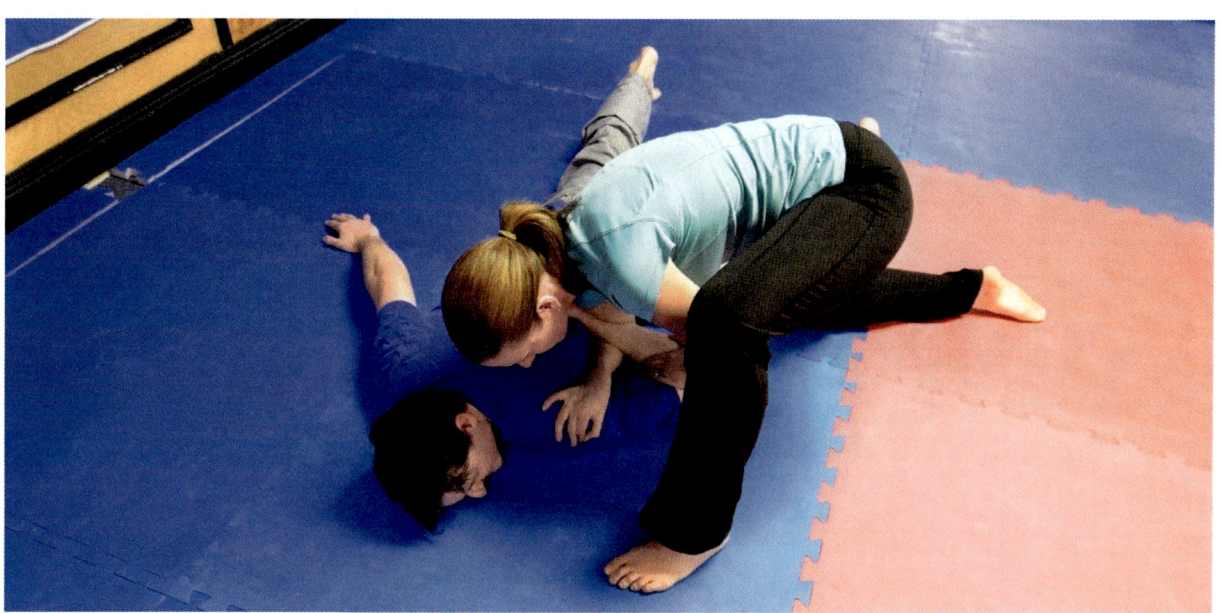

No husbands were harmed in the filming of this exercise.

Chapter 8 – Hokwondo

"I have been a Ho Kwon Do student with the Grand Master for 20 months at this point in time. I have a background in healthcare as a Doctor of Chiropractic for 42 years, 12 years of wrestling as an athlete and a coach, and also six years of Kung Fu training in the 1980's.

When I began training Ho Kwon Do it had been over 25 years since I had participated in any martial arts. I was a little hesitant to begin because of my age at that time being 66 years old, and rusty from not working out at that level. I found Grand Master Kwon to be most welcoming and having me start slow and work my way into shape. I was also impressed about the culture of the school itself with all levels of participants willing to teach and help each other to become better at the art. In my mind that comes from the Grand Master setting the tone that we all respect each other and there is no elitism even among the higher ranks.

I enjoy the lessons the Grand Master teaches not only on Ho Kwon Do but on how to live life healthier and happier. Also, how to use your body effectively during the day to maximize your body functions and motion. I also enjoy his take on the philosophy of the art and how to incorporate that in your daily activities.

I personally have become more physically fit and I incorporate practicing the information on a daily basis to improve my proficiency. I am closing in on 68 years of age, and I feel my work with Grand Master Kwon has helped make me more physically fit and stronger than most people in my age group. I see how smooth and fluid Grand Master Kwon moves and that it is something I work toward attaining for myself."

~ Dr. Thomas R. De Vita

For many, many years I saw that we need a martial art that is better for older people and more practical for self-defense. Hokwondo uses mostly hand techniques, very fast and in combination. The hands strike and come back even before being fully extended to a locked position. The techniques are used in combination with pressure points and joint locks. Because it is designed to be practical, it is also rather dangerous. Hokwondo is designed to stop any opponent, armed or unarmed, very fast. The Hokwondo student uses only as much force as necessary to stop the attacker with a fast combination of punches, pressure points and joint locks.

Hokwondo usually fights from a close distance, arm's length or closer. In Hokwondo, there is no difference between a block and a strike; they are the same action. There is no difference between defense and attack. Attack *is* the defense. The combination of techniques continues to flow without stop until the opponent is finished. The student must be able to attack in any direction and to change direction smoothly without stopping, following the natural flow of energy.

Most real fights end on the ground, so it is important to practice falling. Students learn to fall and roll safely when they practice with each other.

Hokwondo techniques are delivered very fast. To develop skill, the combinations must be practiced over and over until they become an unconscious reflex.

Martial arts use two kinds of power. There is pushing power, to move a big, solid object through force. There is also cracking power, the ability to break an object by striking very fast. Explosives can push large amounts of dirt through pushing power. They can also break steel through cracking power. Hokwondo uses the snap of short, focused strikes delivered rapidly in combination to precise targets in order to disable an opponent.

Strength can be hard or soft. Soft strength is like bamboo that will bend in the wind but not break. Look at the hurricanes that blow over strong buildings while palm trees bend and survive. Soft strength is toughness. It bends a little under stress but survives.

Soft power, or toughness, comes from inner energy, from your life force. For this reason, it is also very important to teach the students how to build *ki gong*, so we do these exercises with every lesson. In Hokwondo, we develop all the basic forms of power: pull, push, twist, lift and snap. The *ki gong* exercises develop all types of power. They also help the student stay healthy even when they grow old.

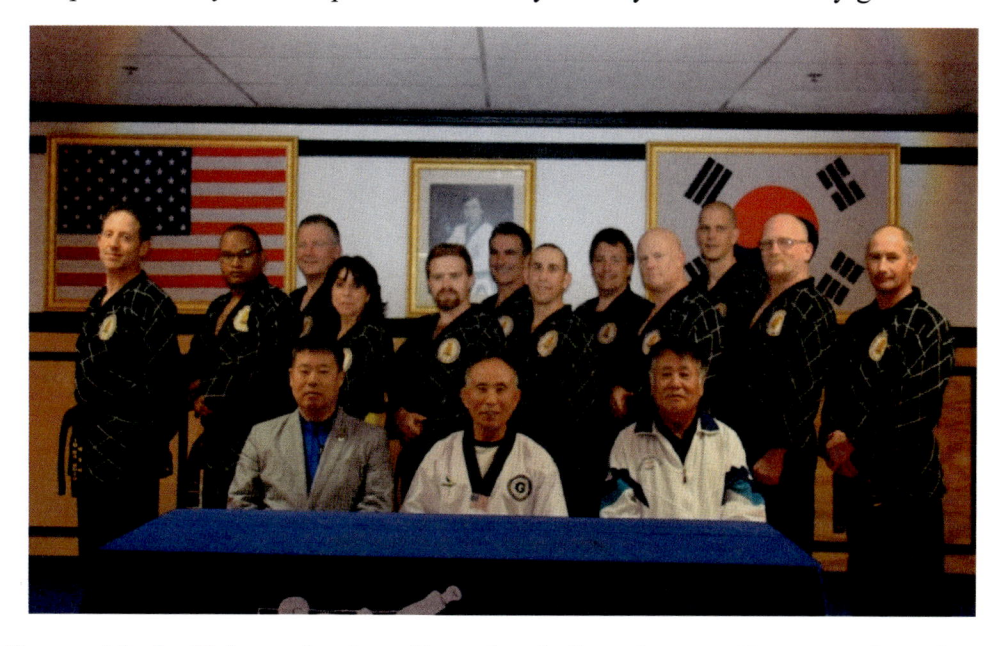

Grandmaster Kwon with the Hokwondo class. Seated with Grandmaster Kwon are Grandmasters Seung Bok Lee (left) and Tae Byung Park (right)

"I started training nine years ago in Hokwondo. At first, I found the basics difficult to remember. With patience and a lot of repetition, it became easier and more enjoyable. One thing I am confident in is that no matter where I am, or how I feel mentally or physically, I can rely on my Hokwondo skills. I don't need to stretch or warm up to be able to use most techniques. The best thing is I feel I do not have to harm anyone to show them the error of their ways. I have no natural inclination to inflict pain on anyone."

~Jerry O'Donoghue
3rd Dan Blackbelt, Hokwondo

Chapter 9 – Decide Now

"Grandmaster Kwon is the one example I can point to of a true grandmaster martial artist. He is humble and modest. He gets up every day and goes to work. Then he does it again and again, over and over."

~ Grandmaster Han D. Cho
Head Instructor, Cornell University Sports Taekwondo Club

Martial arts are about protecting life, so it is important for students to build their own life force to improve their health. In this way, there is no difference between protecting yourself and protecting others. You must help others to help yourself; you must help yourself to help others.

If you have good things inside yourself – love, wisdom, advice – share them with others. By sharing them, you will improve your own health. If you keep everything to yourself and hold them inside, it will lead to bad health and physical deterioration.

Sharing yourself is more important than sharing money or material possessions.

Everything has *um-yang* balance. Male and female, night and day, fire and water, hot and cold, success and failure, good and bad. Everything. But you can change the balance. No one will give you health or success. You must go and get it yourself.

There is no difference between the physical and the mental. Your attitude brings happiness and physical health, so it is important to keep yourself motivated and optimistic. When life brings you something bad or you temporarily fail at your goals, face the bad things and fix them quickly, then leave them behind. Go back to the little things that make you happy. (I like golf. Some people like music. It's your choice.) It is important to stay happy because happiness brings health.

Motivate yourself by saying "I can do it!" It will lead to success. Avoid the negative attitude that says, "I can't do it." It will lead to failure. Kick out the bad energy and bring in the good. It is easier to stay healthy than to get healthy.

So many people by 70 (or even 40!) say, "I'm too old." Don't say that! None of my exercises are big efforts to make big changes all at once. Slapping your body starting with hands, then arms, chest, belly, back, buttocks, back of legs, front of legs up and down, inside and out three or four times only takes a minute or two. These exercises are small, small things you do over and over, day by day that eventually make big changes. Start small and persist. Never give up! Life is a challenge that never ends. There is no final exercise.

Bigger hardship comes from avoiding small hardships. For example, learning to ride a bike involves falling down. If you avoid learning to ride because you don't want to fall, you will never gain the greater skill of riding.

In the same way, big happiness comes through big sadness. The darker the night, the brighter the dawn. The deeper the sadness, the greater the happiness when it comes. Hard times yield great happiness later.

Change is always hard, like getting new clothes or shoes. At first, they are stiff and uncomfortable. But after a while they become comfortable. People are afraid of new ideas in the same way. Facing problems leads to solutions and growth. You need to keep an open mind and believe in yourself. When bad things happen, be grateful for the challenge. Overcome the hardship and good things will come. Trust yourself.

If you are always truthful and pursue justice, you will have peace inside. Keeping a peaceful mind will guard your health. Losing self-control only brings more bad things. Keeping your self-control brings good things later.

The saddest thing is to live without purpose, without hope. Having a goal to give you purpose, no matter what it is, leads to a happy life. Maybe it is a college degree. Maybe it is just your next belt in Taekwondo. Choose a goal and make a plan for your life.

Start taking action today! You can buy exercise equipment, but you can't buy muscles. You can pay for a personal trainer, but you can't buy health. You can buy a book, but not knowledge. You must decide to take action.

Decide now to have a long, happy life!

Korean Terms

Taekwondo – The national martial art of Korea, characterized by its emphasis on head-height kicks, jumping and spinning kicks, and fast kicking techniques

Dojang – Training floor or school where a martial art is practiced

Dobok – Martial arts uniform

Hokwondo – A complete martial art and self-defense system created by Grandmaster Young A. Kwon which utilizes joint locks, pressure points, kicks, hand strikes and blocks. It also uses long-range, short-range and speed techniques.

Kwan Jang Nim – Grandmaster, either 8th or 9th Dan Black Belt in the Taekwondo system of ranks

Dan jun – A point in traditional Chinese and Korean medicine located approximately two finger-widths below the navel in the belly, believed to be a storage place for *qi* or *ki* energy

Poom sae – Formalized series of stances, blocking, striking, and kicking techniques.

Um Yang – Korean equivalent of Yin Yang, the inseparable balance of positive and negative aspects to everything

Kihap – The loud shout when delivering a blow or kick

Because Korean is so different from English, you will often find variations in spelling. The grandmaster is not an English scholar and few of his students have studied Korean. The Korean sounds do not correspond exactly to English letters and there is disagreement on how to form the words. One of the delightful, if occasionally confusing, challenges in writing this book was sorting through the variety of expressions used by the grandmaster and his students. I chose to leave the variations of spelling in place as much as possible in order to preserve the flavor of communication rather than force an artificial standardization onto the text.

~ Lloyd Sparks

About the Authors

Grandmaster Young Ahn Kwon

Grandmaster Young Ahn Kwon is the founder of Kwon's Taekwondo in Tewksbury, Massachusetts as well as the creator of the martial art Hokwondo. He holds the highest rank attainable in Taekwondo, that of Ninth Dan Black Belt. He also holds high ranks in other martial arts. He served in Special Operations in the Marine Corps of the Republic of Korea (ROK).

Grandmaster Kwon was trained in Korean Traditional Medicine and practiced in South Korea until immigrating to the United States in 1987. His knowledge and skill in healthcare and the martial arts uniquely qualify him to speak on this much-neglected subject.

Biography

2005 – 2016	Founded Kwon's Taekwondo, Inc., Lunenburg, Massachusetts.
1989 – Present	Founded Kwon's Taekwondo, Inc., Tewksbury, Massachusetts.
1988 – 1989	Chief Instructor for the United States Army at Fort Devens, Massachusetts.
1987	Chief Instructor for the Korean National Demonstration Team; brought the team to the United States.
1973 – 1975	Completed two-year specialized course at the Tae Kwon Life-Force Remedy Sports Association, Seoul, South Korea for acupuncture and chiropractic medicine; also accomplished in acupressure and sports medicine.
1973 – 1987	Founded Young Ahn's Taekwondo School in Suwon, South Korea.
1969 – 1972	Served in the Republic of Korea Marine Corps (ROKMC).
	Martial Arts Instructor for the Marine Corps.
	Represented the Marine Corps in competitions and trained marine counterparts in the use of high-level, lethal martial arts techniques.
1965 – 1967	Lightweight Asian Kickboxing Champion for 3 years, undefeated.

Ranks and Certifications

World Taekwondo Federation-certified Grandmaster awarded by the Kukkiwon, World Taekwondo Headquarters, Seoul, South Korea.

Moo Duk Kwan 9th Dan Black Belt

Hapkido 9th Dan Black Belt

Muay Thai champion kickboxer

Publications and Articles

Featured in article, "Master is a Medicine Man," in the May, 1993 issue of *Taekwondo Times* magazine.

Featured in article, "Grandmaster & Disciples," in the February, 1999 issue of *World Taekwondo* magazine.

Featured in article "Grandmaster of the Year," in the January, 2012 issue of *Taekwondo Times* magazine.

Featured in article "Grandmaster Young A. Kwon: Family is the Way of Life," in the March, 2015 issue of *Taekwondo Times* magazine.

Professional Memberships

Member of the Kukkiwon International Advisory Committee

Member of the World Taekwondo Federation

Member of the United States Taekwondo Grandmasters Society (Consultative Committee)

New England President of the Pan American Moo Duk Kwan Society

Member of the International Kickboxing Association

Founder of the World Ho Kwon Do Federation

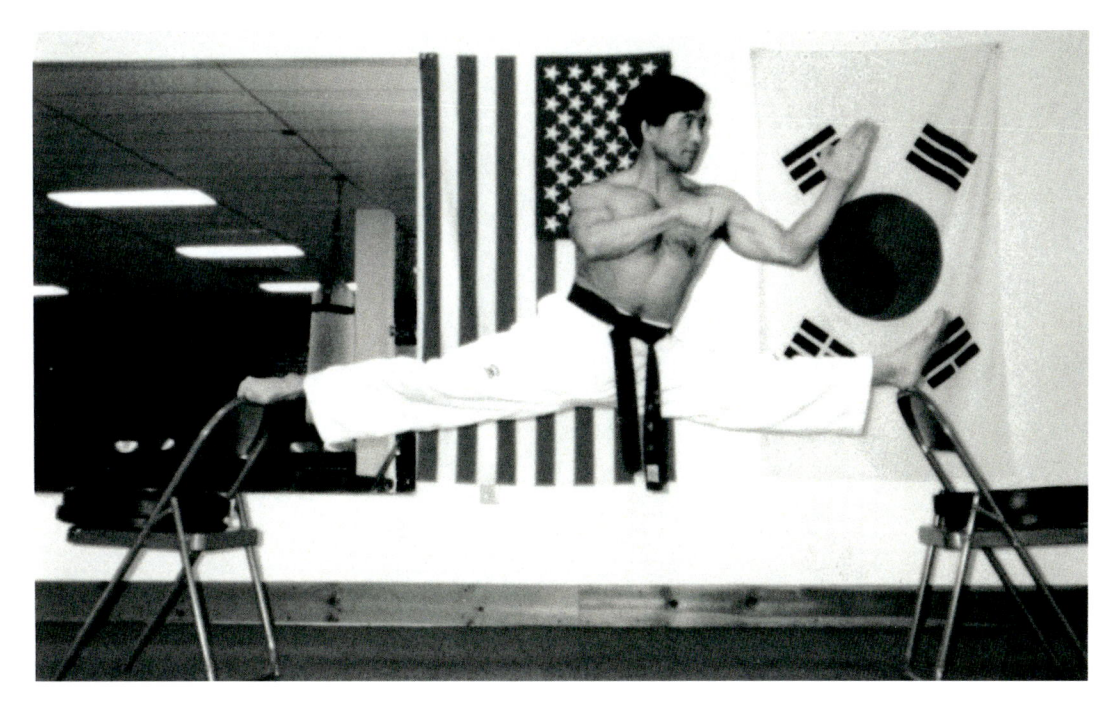

Grandmaster Kwon 1990

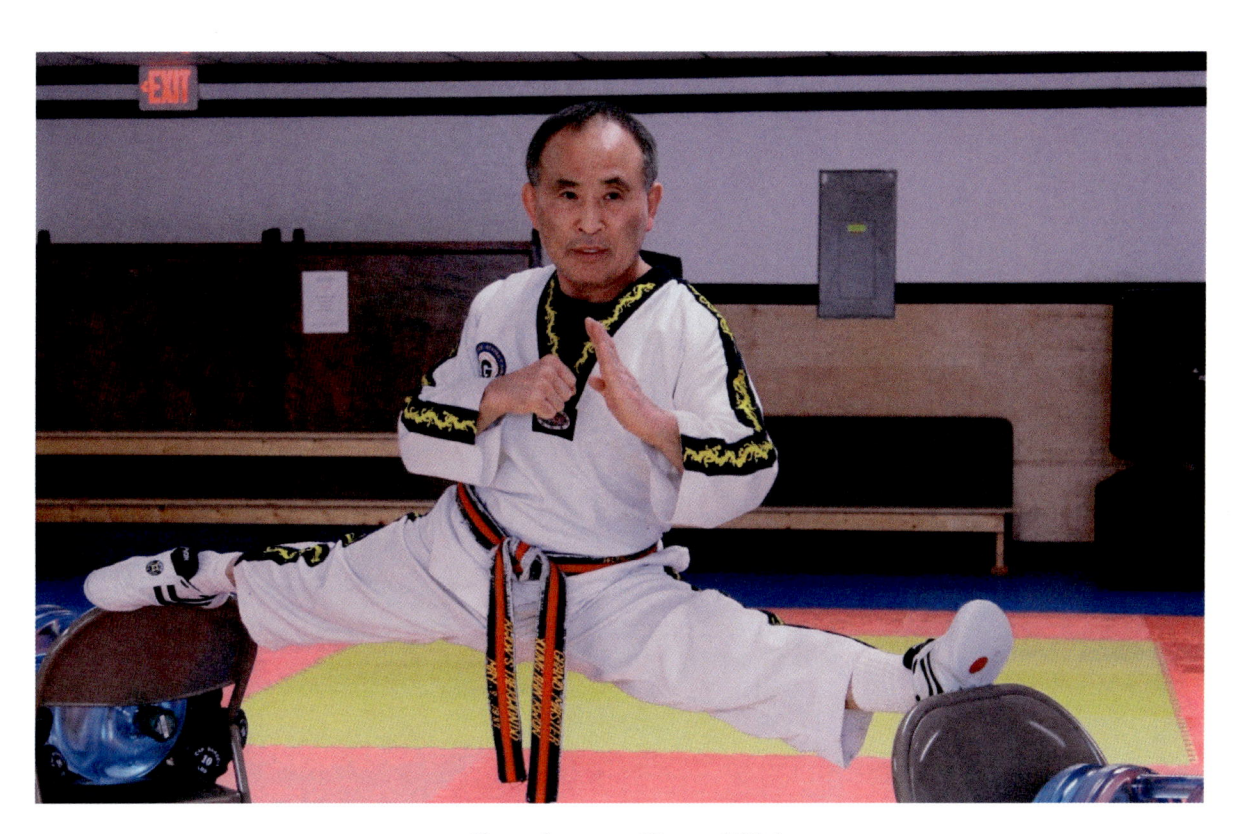

Grandmaster Kwon 2014

Dr. Lloyd Sparks

Lloyd Sparks, MD is a writer, clinician, and researcher. He holds the rank of third dan black belt in Taekwondo and has been a student of Grandmaster Kwon since 2009. He has also studied Chi Kung Fu, Wado Ryu karate, and Brazilian jiujitsu. He served in US Army Special Forces, retiring at the rank of sergeant major in 2012.

Dr. Sparks is certified in Age Management Medicine, Pain Management, and Forensic Medicine. He has a PhD in Biochemistry and has published numerous articles on health and fitness. His formal education also includes chiropractic, nutrition, and massage.

His other works include the award-winning young adult novel *The Uranium Plant*, and the autobiographical *Detour: My Brief but Amusing Career as a Bible Smuggler* and *Boondoggle: My Unexpected Career as a Military Defense Contractor*.

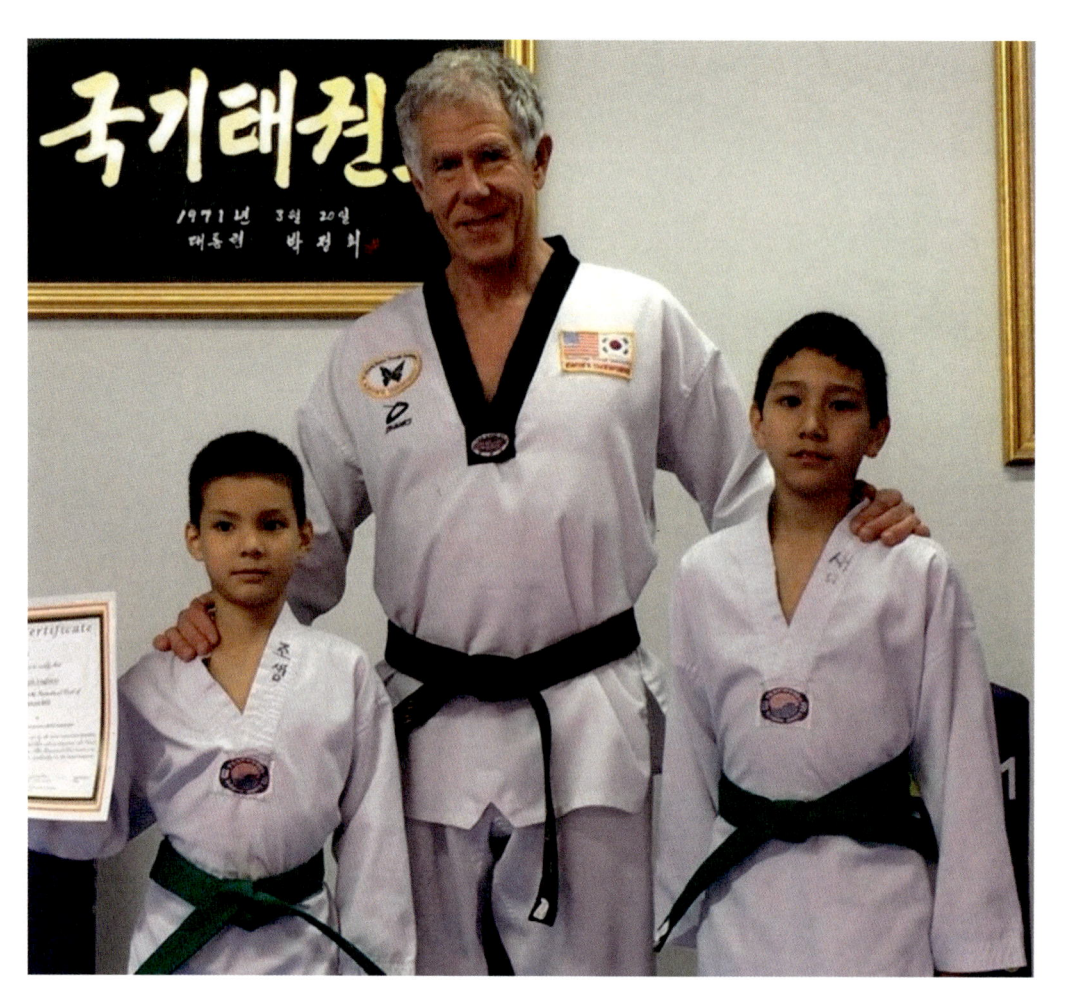

Lloyd Sparks with two young students Joseph and Sam Gagliano

Made in the USA
Middletown, DE
13 August 2019